BASIC SCIENCE FOR ANAESTHETISTS

This is a revised edition of a book originally titled *Anaesthetic Data Interpretation*. The new title better reflects the contents of the book, which contains additional chapters relevant to the Primary FRCA examination. New topics covered include the ventilatory response to oxygen and carbon dioxide, which is now a core knowledge requirement, new concepts in cardiovascular physiology, receptor types and the molecular actions of anaesthetics. Some of the revisions reflect advances in technology; for example, the uses of the capnograph and the oxygen analyser have advanced considerably in recent years. The aim is to provide a concise and understandable review of the physics, mathematics, statistics, physiology and pharmacology of anaesthesia. *Basic Science for Anaesthetists* is a concise and informative text, which will be invaluable for trainee anaesthetists and an aid to teaching for the trainers.

SYLVA DOLENSKA qualified from Charles University, Prague, trained as an anaesthetist in the UK and is currently Consultant Anaesthetist at William Harvey Hospital, Ashford, Kent. She has also acquired the KSS Deanery Certificate in Teaching. Her other key professional interests are airway management and obstetric anaesthesia.

D1459455

BASIC SCIENCE FOR ANAESTHETISTS

BY

SYLVA DOLENSKA MD LMSSA FRCA

Consultant Anaesthetist, Department of Anaesthetics,
The William Harvey Hospital, Ashford, Kent, UK

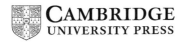
CAMBRIDGE
UNIVERSITY PRESS

CAMBRIDGE UNIVERSITY PRESS

Cambridge, New York, Melbourne, Madrid, Cape Town, Singapore, São Paulo

Cambridge University Press
The Edinburgh Building, Cambridge CB2 2RU, UK

Published in the United States of America by Cambridge University Press, New York

www.cambridge.org
Information on this title: www.cambridge.org/9780521676021

First published 2000 by Greenwich Medical Media Ltd
First published by Cambridge University Press 2006

Printed in the United Kingdom at the University Press, Cambridge

A catalogue record for this publication is available from the British Library

Library of Congress Cataloguing in Publication data

ISBN-13   978-0-521-67602-1 paperback
ISBN-10   0-521-67602-9 paperback

Every effort has been made in preparing this publication to provide accurate and up-to-date information which is in accord with accepted standards and practice at the time of publication. Although case histories are drawn from actual cases, every effort has been made to disguise the identities of the individuals involved. Nevertheless, the authors, editors and publishers can make no warranties that the information contained herein is totally free from error, not least because clinical standards are constantly changing through research and regulation. The authors, editors and publishers therefore disclaim all liability for direct or consequential damages resulting from the use of material contained in this publication. Readers are strongly advised to pay careful attention to information provided by the manufacturer of any drugs or equipment that they plan to use.

Cambridge University Press has no responsibility for the persistence or accuracy of URLs for external or third-party internet websites referred to in this publication, and does not guarantee that any content on such websites is, or will remain, accurate or appropriate.

To my husband

CONTENTS

ABBREVIATIONS and SYMBOLS

Units are shown in parentheses

a	acceleration (m s^{-2})
A	ampere
A	area (m^2)
c	concentration (g l^{-1})
C	compliance (l Pa^{-1})
C	coulomb
Cd	candela
°C	degrees Celsius
d	distance (m)
d	rate of change (derivation)
D	diameter (m)
e	base of natural logarithms
E	extinction coefficient
F	force (kg m per s = N)
g	gram
I	light or current intensity (Cd or A)
J	joule
K or k	constant
K	kelvin
l	length (m)
l	litre
m	metre
mol	amount of substance that contains as many elementary particles as there are atoms in 0.012 kg carbon-12
n	number
N	newton
P	power (J s^{-1} = W)
p	pressure (P_a); see chapter on gas pipeline pressure for other units and their conversion
Pa	pascal
Q	electric charge (C)
$\dot{Q}$	flow (l s^{-1}) (also denoted as dV/dt)
r	radius (m)
R	resistance (Pa l^{-1} per s)
R	universal gas constant
Re	Reynolds' number (dimensionless)
STP	standard temperature and pressure (0 °C, 1 atmosphere = 273 K, 101.3 kPa)
t	time (s)

T	absolute temperature (K)
v	velocity (m s^{-1})
V	volume (1)
W	watt
W	work (kg m^2)

Greek symbols

η (eta)	viscosity
μ (mu)	population mean
π (pi)	3.141592653 ...
ρ (ro)	density
σ (sigma)	population standard deviation (SD)
Σ (capital sigma)	summa = total
τ (tau)	time constant
ζ (zeta)	damping

FIGURE CAPTIONS

FOREWORD

The syllabus for the Primary FRCA examination is broad, covering basic anaesthesia and associated skills together with an in depth knowledge of the principles of basic science which underlie clinical practice. Added to this, is the requirement to pass the examination at an early stage of the trainee's career. Often, it is an inadequate understanding or wariness of concepts which involve physics or simple mathematics that is the impediment to success in the examination.

The author has written a book which explains the principles of physics, mathematics and statistics and applies many of them to an understanding of anaesthetic apparatus, clinical measurement, cardiovascular and respiratory physiology, and general pharmacology. Each concept is supported by a graph or diagram which is explained in the text. A graphical display of data or a good diagram is often the key to interpretation and conveying a thorough understanding of subject matter to an examiner. This approach applies equally when responding to a question in an oral examination or when supplementing a written answer.

This book is undoubtedly aimed at the candidate sitting the Primary examination, however, the Final FRCA candidate should not forget that the theme of questioning in the second oral examination is basic science applied to anaesthesia, intensive care and pain management. This book should not be regarded as a substitute for the standard textbooks but will be invaluable as a supplement and also for revision. Senior colleagues will find in this book a concise refresher course on basic science principles that will be of personal value and will assist in teaching trainees. A proportion of candidates fail the oral section of an examination having done well in the written part. This would suggest they have the knowledge but fail in their verbal presentation. There is a fund of questions, diagrams and graphs in this book that can form the basis of mock vivas for candidates to improve their fluency of presentation in preparation for the examination proper.

Leslie E. Shutt
Bristol
January 2000

FOREWORD

The successful and safe practice of anaesthesia depends, amongst other things, upon a good comprehension of the scientific foundations of the subject. It is for this reason that all examining boards set scientific questions in various parts of their examinations, whether in conventional multiple choice or single best answer format, formal essays, short answers, OSCEs (objective structured clinical examinations) or in the oral examinations. Candidates have much more difficulty with the basic and applied science sections of the examination than with any other parts. In particular, the understanding of physics and the application of physical principles are not easy. Many candidates, quite frankly, lack basic education in these topics when starting at medical school; moreover, they are less easy to learn as one grows older, especially when embarking on a busy clinical career in anaesthesia.

I can remember from my own experiences as a candidate for the Primary FRCA (then called the FFARCS) a legendary examiner who would push a sheet of paper over to the unfortunate candidate during a *viva* and invite him or her to draw the structure of pethidine (merperidine, Demerol). Thank goodness that does not happen nowadays, but reliance on the production of drawings or graphs to illustrate a point is very common, for indeed a good picture is worth a thousand (some say ten thousand) words. The interpretation of radiographs and electrocardiograms has stood the test of time. Moreover, many examiners now rely upon previously produced drawings or photographs - of varying clarity and quality - as part of the examination, and I must confess that I have produced some of my own over the years.

Sylva Dolenska originally intended to use the apt subtitle *"do you get the picture?"* for this book but it was changed to *Anaesthetic Data Interpretation* and the Primary FRCA examination became her target. Nevertheless, success in any examination in anaesthesia, wherever in the world, relies upon the grasp and understanding of basic scientific facts. Hence her approach of using illustrations (linked to explanations) that have almost come straight from the examiner's briefcase provides welcome help for candidates. Examples are drawn from everyday clinical anaesthesia: the use of medical gases, respiratory and circulatory physiology, the behaviour and distribution of drugs, and concluding with concepts of receptors. Many current and future candidates for examinations in anaesthesia should be grateful for the help this will give them.

Anthony P. Adams
Professor of Anaesthetics in the University of London at the Guy's, King's and St. Thomas' School of Medicine, King's College, London.
January 2000

PREFACE

There are many textbooks to chose from when preparing for the FRCA examination; the candidate suffers not from lack of information but rather from being inundated with it. The candidate then has the task of information sorting and data compression to memorize and utilize all this information. Graphic representation of data is an excellent form of data compression; figures or drawings are frequently asked about at the viva examination, particularly since the candidate's understanding of a problem comes across most clearly when drawing a figure or a using a picture. For anaesthetists whose first language is not English, figures are also a good way of approaching a topic – I certainly find it easier to find words when describing a plot.

I constructed parts of this book when revising for the Primary Examination and afterwards when preparing tutorials. The book differs from most in that the text accompanies the pictures, rather than the pictures complementing the text. In many cases, the text is simply a legend to the figure or diagram, expanded by background information. For this reason, the figures are described only by the names of the axes and their units along with identification of any other important lines and symbols. The layout – each page of text opposite the relevant figure(s) – conveys the essential link between picture and text, and I hope it makes orientation and understanding easier.

Not all knowledge required for the FRCA (Primary or Final) is suitable for graphical representation. The properties of anaesthetic drugs, for instance, lend themselves to tabulation rather than to diagrammatic representation, and they require little in the way of understanding of fundamental concepts. I therefore recommend the reader to read basic, comprehensive textbooks *before* beginning this text because, first, this book is not intended as comprehensive and, second, because a complete textbook will give a fuller perspective on the topics represented.

The book was updated according to the latest FRCA syllabus, and it shows the relevance of basic science to clinical anaesthesia in practical examples throughout. A choice had to be made, however, even among the topics suitable for illustration. Most of the topics I have chosen rank highly in order of importance to anaesthetists (Jones, *Anaesthesia* (October 1997), 930). Descriptive statistics and mathematical concepts, although not popular, are included as they appear in the syllabus and because they constitute the basic knowledge on which the candidate can build an understanding of other subjects seen as more relevant to anaesthesia (such as the principles of measurement).

Although the book is intended mainly for the Primary FRCA candidate, it would also make an excellent 'aide-memoire' for clinical tutors and all practising anaesthetists who undertake teaching and wish to remain connected with the basic principles on which anaesthesia is built. I hope the prospective FRCA candidate will find the book useful.

S. D.
October 1999
London

PREFACE TO THE SECOND EDITION

This is a revised edition of the book originally titled *Anaesthetic Data Interpretation*, published by Greenwich Medical Media in 2000. The new title better reflects the contents of the book.

New chapters have been added on the direct or indirect advice of Primary FRCA examiners. Ventilatory response to oxygen and ventilatory response to carbon dioxide are now core knowledge requirements, and form the basis of clinical decision making. New concepts in cardiovascular physiology, such as the end-systolic pressure–volume relationship are important to our understanding of control of cardiac function. The concept of total intravenous anaesthesia has evolved around pharmacokinetic research into how drugs behave when injected at a steady rate. Receptor types and molecular actions of anaesthetics, although may seem far removed from clinical practice, are however part of the examination syllabus, providing wider background which helps to understand how anaesthetics work. Receiver operating characteristic, an idea recently introduced in medical statistics from aviation, is a concept that will help to understand scientific articles.

Basic science does not change but technology does and some of the revisions reflect this. Technical advances in monitoring continue apace. The capnograph and the oxygen analyser are no longer the heavy cumbersome machines that were difficult to maintain. It is important to know how these machines work, in order to understand what problems may arise and to troubleshoot.

Updated chapters are based on contemporary texts and new concepts which are now contained in the syllabus. Many chapters have been improved with additions of new diagrams.

The text is fairly didactic and describes mostly what is usual, or what the usual deviation from norm is, since this would be the expectation at the Primary FRCA examination.

The second edition is still slimline and I hope it will continue as a useful aid to learning for trainee anaesthetists.

SD, Ashford 2005

Part 1

Physics, mathematics, statistics, anaesthetic apparatus

Gas compression, relationship of volume, pressure and temperature

The **universal gas equation** describes the equation of state for 1 mole ideal gas:

$$p\,V = R\,T,$$

where R = molar (universal) gas constant = $N_A.k$ (Avogadro and Boltzman constants).

The simple equation expresses three different ideal gas laws, depending on which variable is chosen to be constant (and therefore taken out of the equation). The assumption for an ideal gas is that the molecules do not occupy any space; this clearly is not true in practice.

In Figure 1, all three gas laws are depicted. The individual curves (rectangular hyperbolas) relate to **Boyle's law**: they show the relationship between pressure and volume when temperature is constant – pressure and volume are inversely related. Each curve shows the relationship for a certain temperature, and therefore is called an **isotherm**. The crosses relate to **Charles' law**: when pressure is constant, the volume is directly proportional to temperature. The dots illustrate **Gay–Lussac's law**: when volume is constant, pressure is directly proportional to temperature.

Avogadro's hypothesis states that the number of molecules per unit volume is independent of the gas concerned, at a given temperature and pressure. At standard temperature and pressure (STP) it is 6.022×10^{23} molecules in 22 litres (Avogadro's number). This number of molecules is equal to 1 mole gas. This means that 1 mole of a gas, allowed to expand until it reaches equilibrium with atmospheric pressure, will expand to fill a volume of 22 litres. Conversely, the **pressure exerted** by a **given number of molecules** of ideal gas in a **given volume** and **temperature** is constant (6.022×10^{23} molecules in 22 litres will exert a pressure of 1 atmosphere) and is **independent of its molecular weight**. For an illustration, see Figure 2, the molecules, heavy or light, are floating in the given space; the number of molecules and the average distance between them is the same. Random thermal movement of heavier molecules will be less at a given temperature than that of lighter molecules; the resulting kinetic energy will be the same, and so will be the pressure inside the container.

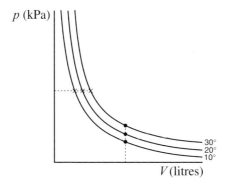

Figure 1. Three gas laws: Boyle's, Charles' and Gay–Lussac.

WITHDRAWN

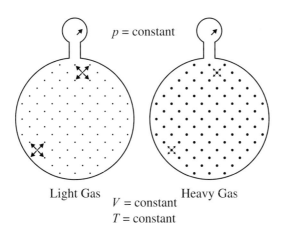

Figure 2. Avogadro's hypothesis.

Real gas compression

Forces of adhesion in the gas lessen the impact on the container. The result is that the pressure measured is less than that predicted by the universal gas equation. The effect is magnified in a smaller volume.

Also, the molecules are not negligible in size; their total volume lessens the volume of the container, decreasing the distance of travel; a correction for the volume of the molecules (V_o) has to be applied.

When gas is compressed at a sufficiently low temperature, the forces of adhesion eventually cause its liquefaction (i.e. the forces of attraction overcome the random thermal motion).

Isothermic compression – decompression

Figure 3 shows slow compression of nitrous oxide under various temperature conditions. Because compression is slow, there is sufficient time for temperature equilibration with the surroundings. This pressure–volume change is called **isothermic**.

The top isotherm for 50 °C behaves as an ideal gas isotherm. At 36.5 °C the isotherm just touches the lightly shaded area in the graph, which represents the gas and liquid phase. This temperature is the **critical temperature** of nitrous oxide, above which the **gas cannot be liquefied** at any pressure. At lower temperatures, here 20 °C, the gas can be liquefied. If compression is slow to allow temperature to remain constant, the pressure in the container remains constant until all gas is liquefied: the decrease in volume of the container is matched by a decrease in volume of the gaseous phase (which is now called vapour) as it is being liquefied. The space above the liquid phase is saturated with the vapour, and the pressure inside the container at the given temperature is the **saturated vapour pressure** (which is constant at a given temperature).

Once the total contents are liquefied, and if compression is continued, the pressure inside the container rises steeply, as liquids are virtually incompressible. Slow decompression would follow the same isotherm in the opposite direction.

The phenomenon of liquefaction is used in practice to increase the amount of substance in a container: nitrous oxide can be liquefied at ambient temperature in a moderate climate (but not in the tropics); by contrast, oxygen, with a critical temperature of −119 °C, has to be liquefied in special insulated vessels to prevent its warming.

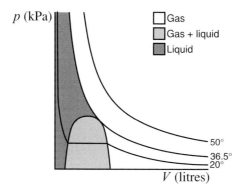

Figure 3. Isothermic compression.

Adiabatic compression – decompression

Figure 4 shows a sudden decompression of a real gas. As the gas suddenly expanded from volume V_1 to volume V_2, thermal energy was lost but time did not allow it to regain heat from the surroundings. The gas therefore moved from its position on the higher isotherm to the lower one; this abrupt pressure–volume change is called **adiabatic**. After reaching temperature equilibrium, the system returned to the original isotherm (from pressure p_2 to pressure p_3).

Anaesthetists using nitrous oxide cylinders can observe both phenomena. Starting with a full cylinder, the pressure at first hardly changes as the vapour is used. The system is on the flat part of the liquid/vapour area of Figure 3; vapour being released from the container is immediately substituted by the formation of more vapour from the liquid phase. Any pressure drop in the cylinder is due to energy loss from the liquid phase because of the latent heat of vaporization, and the system moves onto a lower isotherm. The cylinder starts frosting at its base.

Once all the liquid phase is used up, if using high flow, adiabatic decompression takes place as the pressure inside starts decreasing noticeably and at a higher rate than expected (Figure 4). When the cylinder is turned off, temperature can equilibrate with the ambient air and the gas inside moves back onto a higher isotherm, with the result that the pressure gauge now gives a higher reading because a warmer gas exerts a higher pressure.

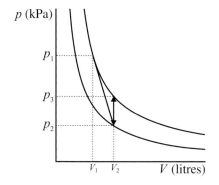

Figure 4. Adiabatic decompression.

Flow and resistance

Flow is defined as the volume of gas or liquid passing a cross sectional area per unit of time. If the volume in a cylinder (or a large tube) is given by the product of its area and length, then the flow in this tube can be thought of as area multiplied by the velocity (see Figure 5):

$$V = A.\ell$$
$$Q = dV/dt = A.d\ell/dt = A.v \qquad \text{(equation 1)}$$

Laminar flow

In laminar flow the fluid moves in a steady manner without eddies or turbulence. A slowly flowing river in a straight stretch is a good approximation. You may notice that the flow near a river bank is very slow while in the centre it is the fastest. This is because of frictional forces between the flow and the side. The speed, or **velocity**, is therefore related to the distance from the side. In fact it can be shown that the maximum velocity is directly proportional to the **square of the radius**; mean velocity is half the maximum velocity ($\bar{v} = v_{max}/2$).

The following are factors affecting the **flow velocity**:

- **Square of the radius**, as mentioned above.
- **Pressure gradient** between the beginning and the end point (a mountain river with a steeper gradient flows much faster than a river near the sea where the gradient is less).
- **Viscosity**: we know from experience that more viscous fluids (e.g. oil) flow more slowly than less viscous fluids (e.g. water). Viscosity in physics is denoted by the Greek 'η' (eta).
- **Length** of the tube: friction slows down the flow at the sides of the tube. The longer the tube, the longer acting the frictional force becomes and the slower the flow.

Mathematically expressed:

$$v \propto r^2$$
$$v \propto \Delta P$$
$$v \propto 1/\ell$$
$$v \propto 1/\eta.$$

From equation 1, this equation has been derived for laminar flow:

$$\dot{Q} = A.\bar{v}$$

where

$$\bar{v} = \frac{\Delta P r^2}{8\eta\ell} \text{ (the factors above and a numerical factor of 8 are}$$

not derived here)

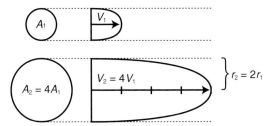

Figure 5. Laminar flow as the product of area and velocity. The influence of doubling the radius on flow.

and

$$A = \pi r^2.$$

Therefore, substitution for area and average velocity gives:

$$\dot{Q} = \frac{\pi r^2 . \Delta P r^2}{8\eta \ell} = \frac{\Delta P \pi r^4}{8\eta \ell}.$$ (equation 2)

This is the **Hagen–Poiseuille** equation that describes laminar flow.

From this we can see that the **radius influences the flow** by its **fourth power**. This is because, as shown above, altering the radius alters both the area and the velocity, which are the determinants of flow, and each is related to the radius by its square function.

When looking at a given tube of fixed radius and length, and passing a flow of a certain fluid of given viscosity, the only variable that remains in the equation is pressure difference: the greater the pressure, the faster the flow – they are directly proportional (see Figure 6). All the other factors (radius, length, viscosity plus the numerical factors) are **fixed** for the given tube and fluid, independent of flow (see Figure 7), and this combination of factors is known as the **resistance** of the tube. We know from experience that flow and resistance are inversely proportional; resistance then becomes the denominator in the Hagen–Poiseuille equation:

$$\dot{Q} = \Delta P / R$$

and therefore, by substitution from equation 2

$$R = \frac{8\eta \ell}{\pi r^4}$$

It can be seen if we wish to alter the resistance to flow, the most influential factor is the radius of the tube: doubling the radius of a tube will reduce the resistance (increase the flow) 16 times (2^4). The length is inversely related to the flow but only by a power of 1. Therefore 'short and thick does the trick'.

The markings on the Rotameter are of unequal length for different flow rates. At low flows the resistance of the orifice around the bobbin behaves according to the Hagen–Poiseuille formula. At high flows it becomes a function of the flow, as the flow becomes turbulent.

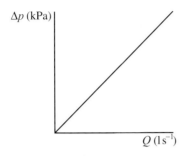

Figure 6. Laminar flow – linear relationship between pressure and flow.

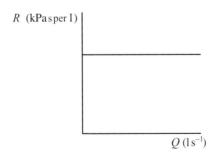

Figure 7. Laminar flow – resistance is independent of flow.

Turbulent flow

If laminar flow passes through a constriction, it changes to turbulent flow; the manner of flow is no longer smooth, but it forms eddies. Now there is no difference in fluid velocity across the tube (i.e. between the flow at the side and the centre of flow), as there was in laminar flow. The **velocity** in the constriction is **increased** overall (as the same amount of fluid has to pass through a narrower tube portion). An example of this can be found on a mountain river reaching a narrow gorge. Because of the lateral movement in eddies, **friction** is a lot greater; the **resistance** to the flow therefore is **no longer constant**. It now depends on the flow: the friction is greater, the greater the speed, i.e. the greater the flow. When measuring resistance in turbulent flow (e.g. during breathing), the flow rate therefore has to be specified.

Also, because of the lateral movement in eddies, flow is no longer directly proportional to the pressure difference; some of the velocity (which, of course, is increased overall) is wasted on the sideways movement, and it can be shown that the flow is now related to **the square root of the pressure difference** as shown in Figure 8 (to double the flow, pressure difference has to be quadrupled).

Usually, the ordinate and abscissa are reversed, so that the pressure difference becomes the dependent variable, and the familiar parabola is vertically orientated. Because resistance is now related to flow, it too becomes a square-root function of the pressure difference (see Figure 9).

Other factors that affect turbulent flow are:

- **Radius**: flow is proportional to its square (not to the fourth power as before), i.e. an increase in flow with a greater diameter is less easily achieved.
- **Length** of tube – an inverse relationship remains.
- **ρ – fluid density** (because it is density that maintains the momentum of the lateral out of stream movement).

Turbulence (the lateral movement), apart from density, is encouraged by higher velocity (also higher momentum), tube diameter, D (more lateral space) and lower viscosity (laminar flow streams less adherent). This is mathematically expressed as the **Reynold's number**, Re:

$$\text{Re} = D.v.\rho/\eta.$$

When Re > 2000 (note it is **dimensionless** as the various units cancel each other out), turbulence occurs. For a given gas, this depends on flow velocity and tube diameter. In severe upper respiratory tract obstruction (e.g. tracheal compression), flow may be improved by providing an inspired mixture of oxygen and helium: because of the low density of helium, the Reynold's number may be reduced sufficiently to convert turbulent flow through the constriction into laminar flow.

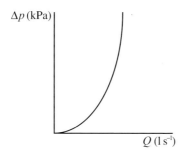

Figure 8. Turbulent flow: driving pressure is the square function of target flow.

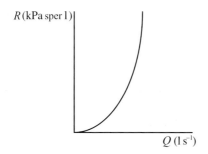

Figure 9. Turbulent flow: resistance is the square function of flow.

1 Heat, vaporization and humidification

Heat is one form of energy; temperature is a measure of the random thermal movement of molecules or atoms (the thermal state of a substance).

Physical changes occur in substances when their temperature is changed by the addition or removal of heat. These are due to increased or reduced thermal movement of molecules.

With progressive addition of heat, **change of phase** happens (from solid to liquid, from liquid to vapour) as cohesive forces are overcome by random thermal movement. The heat necessary to overcome the cohesive forces during change of phase is called latent heat. According to the first law of thermodynamics, substances with a higher temperature (higher thermal state) will pass their heat onto substances with a lower temperature (lower thermal state). Accordingly, to convert a substance from one phase into another, latent heat must be supplied or removed.

Specific latent heat refers to 1 kg of a substance converted from one phase to another at a constant temperature. Temperature and substance must be stated as specific latent heat is temperature-dependent, and each substance has different thermal properties. Water is a liquid at $0\,°C$ and vaporizes at $100\,°C$ at atmospheric pressure (see Figure 10). At higher pressures it would vaporize at higher temperatures, until it reached its critical temperature (data not shown); at this point the specific latent heat is zero. Nitrous oxide is a gas at atmospheric pressure; it must be compressed to liquefy. To turn it back into gas, latent heat of vaporization must be supplied (see the chapter on real gas compression). Figure 11 shows that specific latent heat of nitrous oxide is much higher than that of water at $0\,°C$ but it decreases quickly to zero at $36.5\,°C$, the critical temperature of nitrous oxide.

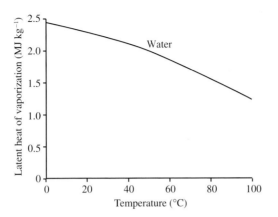

Figure 10. Latent heat of vaporization of water. Reproduced with permission from Butterworth-Heinemann.

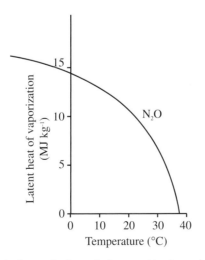

Figure 11. Latent heat of vaporization of nitrous oxide. Reproduced with permission from Butterworth-Heinemann.

Humidification requires addition of latent heat. During inhalation, ambient air is warmed and humidified in the upper airway; latent heat must be supplied for this. During exhalation, the expired gas is cooled in the upper airway and some, but not all, of the heat and water is returned to the nasal mucosa. Because ambient air is usually cooler and less humid than expired air, water and heat from the body are lost during breathing (about 250 ml water and 350 calories per day). The biggest part of heat thus lost is the latent heat of vaporization.

The amount of vapour present in air is limited by temperature. When air contains the maximum amount of vapour, it is said to be **saturated** by it. Figure 12 shows the relationship between temperature and the maximum amount of water vapour in the air. The shape of the line is a parabola but note that it does not go through zero on the y-axis. Notice that at 20 °C, the air contains a smaller mass of water than at 37 °C.

Vaporization

Anaesthetic vaporizers are designed to produce a concentration of anaesthetic vapour that corresponds to the vaporizer setting regardless of gas flow passing through them. The gas in the vaporizer chamber is fully saturated with anaesthetic vapour, but the amount of vapour depends on temperature, as shown above: as the anaesthetic vapour is removed from the vaporizer chamber by the dry gases, latent heat is removed from the remaining liquid and the vaporizer walls. Unless temperature compensation is applied, the amount of vapour and its saturated vapour pressure would drop, as would the vaporizer output. Modern vaporizers have several sophisticated methods of temperature compensation, based on a temperature-controlled valve which adjusts the splitting ratio: as temperature inside the vaporizer decreases, more gas is allowed to pass through the vaporizing chamber to compensate for the loss of saturated vapour pressure. At 20 °C saturated vapour pressure of desflurane is higher than that of most agents. However, because of its low lipid solubility, it has a fairly high minimum alveolar concentration. The vaporizer, therefore, has to be heated to produce sufficient amounts of vapour.

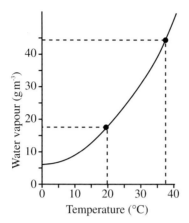

Figure 12. Water vapour content (absolute humidity) of air fully saturated with water, as a function of temperature. Reproduced with permission from Butterworth-Heinemann.

Simple mechanics 1: mass, force, pressure

Mass is a fundamental quantity; the other above-mentioned mechanical quantities are derived from it. Its unit, 1 kilogram, is a basic SI (Système Internationale) unit. Mass means 'quantity of matter'. This description is more or less a tautology; it shows the difficulty in defining the fundamental. Our perception of mass is that of weight, or of an object's opposition to an attempt to move it, which means applying force. In physics, weight in fact is a **force**, defined as the product of **mass and acceleration:** F = m.a. Its unit is 1 newton (N) or 1 kg m per s^2. The gravitational pull is the same in most places on Earth, and gives all objects an acceleration of 9.81 m per s^{-2}. Thus weight is directly proportional to mass, and the two quantities are interchangeable. The kilogram is therefore used as a unit of weight, instead of newton, which is the correct unit. The relationship between mass and weight can be readily demonstrated on weighing scales: 1 kg of mass placed on one side of the scale produces a force (weight) of 9.81 newtons. Consequently, when training operating department assistants, to exert a force of 20 to 40 newtons (for the application of cricoid pressure), the weight they should be aiming for on the scales is 2 to 4 kg. If the legendary apple, which struck Sir Isaac Newton's head as it fell off the tree, weighed approximately 100 grams, it would have struck with a force of about 1 newton.

We know from experience, when pushing an object such as a car or a full supermarket trolley from a stationary position, the greatest force has to be applied before the object starts moving, i.e. gains acceleration. Minimal force is required to keep it moving at a constant velocity (acceleration is zero, force is just sufficient to overcome friction). When stopping, force from the opposite direction has to be applied (i.e. braking) to achieve deceleration.

Pressure is defined as a **force per unit area** $p = F/A$. Its unit is 1 pascal (Pa), equal to 1 N m^{-2}. Because 1 newton is a small force and 1 m^2 is a fairly large area, 1 pascal is a tiny unit of pressure. Force can then be thought of as a product of pressure and area ($F = p.A$). A reciprocal relationship exists between pressure and area for a constant force as shown in Figure 13.

In Figure 14, a constant force is applied to a small and then a large syringe. The flow from the small syringe (point B, Figure 13) is visibly higher (flow being related to the pressure exerted), i.e. syringe emptying is easier than with the large syringe (point A, Figure 13).

During intravenous induction of anaesthesia, constant rate of injection (flow), and therefore constant pressure on the syringe plunger is required. A greater force must be applied to a large syringe with a large cross-sectional area. Anybody who attempted to push fluid out of a 50 ml syringe remembers the aching hand afterwards.

1

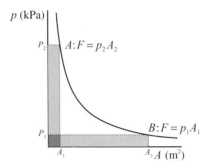

Figure 13. Force as a product of pressure and area; reciprocal relationship between pressure and area for constant force.

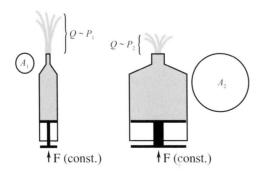

Figure 14. Pressure generated in different size syringes with constant force.

In anaesthetics, the principle of balancing forces is used in **pressure reducing valves**, where high and low pressure gas push against a large area of a diaphragm connected to a rod, as shown in Figure 15. The sum of these forces is opposed by the tension of a spring attached to the other side of the diaphragm. This is set slightly above the force of the high pressure gas acting on the rod. When low gas pressure decreases, the tension of the spring overcomes the forces produced by the gas and the rod is pushed out, opening the high pressure gas inlet. Low pressure then rises sufficiently inside the valve to overcome the tension of the spring and high pressure gas inlet is shut, and the cycle is repeated as low pressure gas escapes.

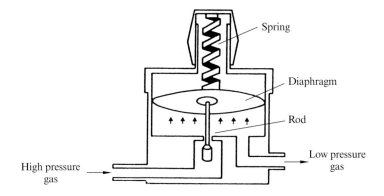

Figure 15. Pressure-reducing valve. Reproduced with kind permission from Butterworth-Heinemann.

1

Simple mechanics 2: work and power

Work is the product of force acting along a distance: $W = F.l$. Its unit is 1 joule (J), equal to 1 N m, which equals 1 kg.m^2 per s^2.

Doing work can be visualised as moving an object using a certain force from one place to another; the force which contributes to the work is in the direction of the movement. The work involved is the product of the force used and the distance between the two places. Reciprocal relationship between force and distance for constant amount of work applies. This reciprocal relationship is used in practice in simple **mechanical devices** to save force: a **ramp** was used by the ancient Egyptians to move some giant stone blocks up the pyramid. The longer the ramp, the less force was needed to push a block up to the same height (pushing an object up a steep slope against gravity needs greater force, and therefore is more exhausting). In Figure 16, the rectangular hyperbola is the line of equal work **(isoerg)**. The points chosen on the line illustrate that for a distance n-times longer, the force used is n-times smaller to make the same amount of work.

When doing **work**, we expend **energy**; work is in fact equivalent to energy, hence the other non-SI unit of energy – kilocalorie (kcal). Thermal energy, kinetic energy, potential energy are all forms of energy; they can change from one form to another but the total energy remains the same. All work can be converted to thermal energy, for instance frictional force in breaking is dissipated as heat. The conversion in the other direction (from thermal energy to work) is also possible but not all heat can thus be converted to work.*) By substitution for force from the pressure formula we obtain:

$$W = F l = p A l = p V$$

The product of area and length is called the volume (e.g. the volume of syringe is the product of its cross-sectional area and the length of the barrel).

In other words, **work** can also be defined as the **product of pressure and volume**. Boyle's law, isothermic compression of ideal gas, is an example of this formula: $p V = $ constant (thermal state, or energy, is the equivalent of work here). The example in Figure 17 shows how compressed gas from a cylinder is used to fill a number of balloons. At point A the volume of gas is low but pressure high. When balloons are filled at point B, the total volume of gas is high but the pressure is lower.

Pumps generate pressures and displace volumes; their work is best defined in terms of these parameters.

---

* **First low** (the law of conservation of energy) **and second law of thermodynamics**, which deals with entropy, are beyond the scope of this book.

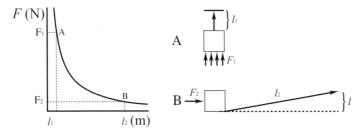

Figure 16. Work as the product of force and distance; reciprocal relationship of force and distance for constant work.

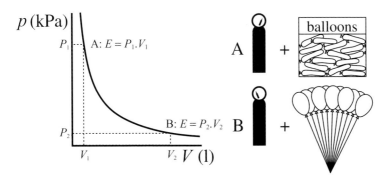

Figure 17. Work (energy) as the product of pressure and volume, reciprocal relationship of pressure and volume for constant energy.

Power is the **rate at which work is done**: $P = dW/dt$. The unit is 1 watt (W), equal to $1\,J\,s^{-1}$. Unfortunately, the symbol for work and for the unit of power is the same letter (W). The symbol d means change, or derivative, that is what increment in work was done in a given time. Derivatives are dealt with in more detail in the chapter on flow measurement. Notice that whilst work has a lot to do with force, time becomes an important factor when dealing with power.

If the force used in some work is constant, by substituting the product $F.l$ for work we obtain:

$$P = F.dl/dt = F.v \text{ (in words, } \textbf{power is the product of force}$$
and velocity).

Imagine a pump worked at a constant pressure to shift fluid, then by substituting pressure and volume for work we obtain $P = dW/dt = p\,dV/dt = p.Q$ (in words, **power is the product of pressure and flow**. From the above formulae, it can be seen that there are three ways of expressing power. Applied to the heart muscle, these will be:

- power as the **slope of the 'work curve'** against time (see Figure 18). If cardiac work is plotted against the systolic ejection time, the slope of the resulting line is steeper for the heart driven by inotropes. Note that the plot would resemble the Starling curve but the parameters are different.
- power as the **product of force and velocity**: this is relevant to the isolated **papillary muscle** preparation. The **force of its contraction and the velocity of the contraction**, as measured in the experimental situation, define the power. Initially, the muscle is stretched to a starting tension F_o, and the velocity is zero. The muscle is then stimulated and as it contracts, the passive stretch is lost and velocity increases. In Figure 19, muscle shortening velocity is plotted against the initial passive stretch (tension). Papillary muscle power, the product of the force and velocity of contraction is the shaded area under the force-velocity line. The force-velocity line is an approximation; force and velocity of contraction are reciprocally related i.e. the line should in theory by a rectangular hyperbola. The graph shows how the area would increase with increased preload (greater initial stretch, higher initial tension but the same maximum velocity), and with increased inotropy (higher initial tension and higher maximum velocity, much higher power).
- power as the **product of pressure and flow: cardiac power** is then a **product of mean blood pressure** and **cardiac output** (see the relevant chapter). Under normal conditions blood pressure and cardiac output are directionally proportional to each other (assuming the aortic impedance Z is constant). In Figure 20 the plot of blood pressure as a function of cardiac output for our purposes is a linear relationship ($p = ZQ$). The slope of this line is the impedance, and the cardiac power is the shaded area under it. Notice that the x-axis here is not the time axis.

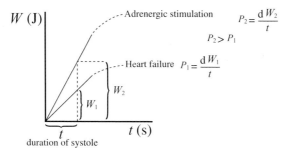

Figure 18. Power as a derivative of work; cardiac power at the two levels of inotropy.

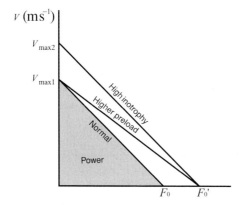

Figure 19. Cardiac power as a product of force and velocity.

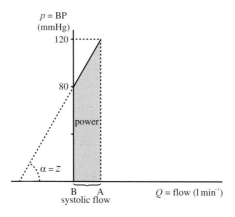

Figure 20. Cardiac power as a product of pressure and flow.

Mathematical concepts

Graphs show relationships between the depicted variables. If this relationship follows a certain rule, or law, then the graph of that relationship will show a certain pattern, which can be described by a formula. The x-axis is sometimes described as the abscissa, and the y-axis as the ordinate.

The linear relationship

$y = k.x$ is the simplest example of a linear relationship. When plotting this on a graph, we could calculate y for several x's, plot each as a point and then join them by a line. We know that this line will be a straight line passing through zero, with a slope α proportionate to k (see Figure 21). If we wished to obtain the sum of all y's for their respective x's up to X, this would be given as the area of triangle XYO, otherwise known as the area under the line k, and the process of obtaining this area is called integration. More on integrals in the chapter on flow measurement.

Rectangular hyperbola

An inverse, or **reciprocal relationship**, $y = k/x$, is depicted by a rectangular hyperbola, k being a constant. $y = 1/x$ is a specific form of this relationship when $k = 1$. The line representing this function is symmetrical across an axis passing through zero at 45°. It asymptotically approaches (never quite reaches) both axes, i.e. neither x nor y can be zero. The reciprocal relationship of y and x is illustrated by looking at rectangles drawn from any point on the hyperbola whose sides are the coordinates of that point: they all have the same area, which is also equal to the area of the square drawn at the intersection of the hyperbola with the 45° axis. In Figure 22 several hyperbolas are drawn, each for a different k, which is the product of y and x (area of the rectangles formed by the coordinates) as shown above. There are numerous examples in anaesthetic practice of variables that are the product of other variables; in particular Boyle's law (the thermal state of ideal gas as a product of its pressure and volume), or end-tidal CO_2 concentration as a product of minute ventilation and fresh gas flow during controlled ventilation in a T-piece (see the appropriate chapters). The relationship of drug dose and effect plotted on a linear scale also produces a rectangular hyperbola but the hyperbola is rising, i.e. it is inverted against the x-axis and shifted up to be above it: $y = a - k/x$ (see the chapter on pharmacodynamics).

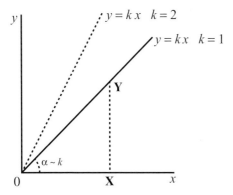

Figure 21. Linear relationship.

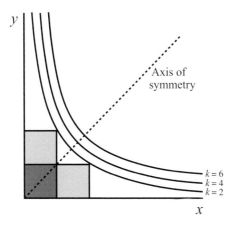

Figure 22. Reciprocal relationship – the rectangular hyperbola.

Parabola

The parabola is the graphical representation of the square function $y = k.x^2$, in anaesthetic practice we come across this shape when considering pressure and flow, or resistance and flow under turbulent flow conditions. In laminar flow, the velocity of the flow is a square function of the tube's radius, while the cross-sectional area is also a square function of the radius. Hence laminar flow is related to the radius by its fourth power (see the chapter on flow). Figure 23 shows two typical examples for two values of K.

Sinusoid waveform

The sine wave is familiar to all who know about alternating current. The graph is a vertical **oscillatory movement** plotted **against time**. The formula is $y = k \sin x$. The wave repeats itself in **cycles** with identical waveforms; its characteristics are **amplitude** (maximum y) and **frequency**. The frequency of repetition is reciprocal to the length of each cycle. A shift of the waveform along the horizontal axis is called a phase shift; at $x = 0$, y will not be zero (the waveform 'starts' mid-cycle).

If two oscillatory movements were added up, the amplitude, frequency or both characteristics of the resulting wave would change. For example, exactly reciprocal waves (the sine wave and its mirror image across the horizontal axis) would cancel each other out, two waves of same frequency and orientation would increase the amplitude, while waves of different frequencies would add up in a more complicated manner, altering the resulting frequency and shape of the waveform (see Figure 24). A sine wave of double the frequency plotted with the original waveform completes two cycles over the time in which the original waveform completed just one cycle. The faster frequency is called the second harmonic (it runs 'in harmony' with the original wave-form, i.e. there is no phase shift). Breaking down of complex waveforms to their fundamental waveforms, the harmonics, is the basis of **Fourier analysis**. Any complex waveform can be broken down into its sine wave components; rounded waveforms contain a smaller number of harmonics while spikes consist of a large number of high-frequency components. For instance, analysis of aortic pressure waveform produces 10 harmonics, an electrocardiogram contains up to 50 harmonics of frequency range 1–100 Hz and intracardiac electrical potentials contain 400 high-frequency harmonics.

A measuring apparatus following an oscillatory movement can only be accurate if its frequency response matches the highest frequency contained in the waveform (see the chapter on electromanometers).

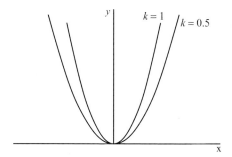

Figure 23. Square function – parabola.

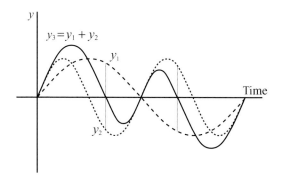

Figure 24. Sine waves and their addition.

Exponentials 1: the curves

Exponential growth (e.g. chain reaction, growth of bacteria)

An exponential is a power by which we raise a number. General exponential growth formula is:

$$y = b^x.$$

The graph of exponential growth (Figure 25a) represents the formula $y = 2^x$. The value of y never can be zero, as it is a number (b) to the power of another number (x). When $x = 0, y = 1$ because any number to the power of zero $= 1$ (n^0 is the same as n^x/n^x). Apart from the variable x, the exponent (power) can also have a fixed component. For exponential growth, this constant exponent is called the growth rate constant; it can be any number except zero, i.e. it can be a fraction. The formula then becomes

$$y = b^{k.x}$$

where k is the growth rate constant. (Note: $y = x^2$, i.e. the square function is a different shape – parabola, and it goes through 0.)

The bacterial growth graph (Figure 25b) represents the formula $y = 2^{t/20}$. The x-axis became in this example the time axis, and doubling time of the bacteria is 20 min. The growth rate constant is 0.05, or $^1/_{20}$. The negative part of the x-axis is not shown. This is because in physiological processes we are interested in their time-course from time zero; what happened before time zero usually does not conform to the exponential curve, but after time zero, the starting point, it does.

Exponential decay (e.g. drug elimination, decrease of transmitted light intensity with distance)

Decay being the reverse of growth, the sign changes and so does the orientation of the curve; it is inverted around the y-axis. The mathematical formula is:

$$y = b^{-x}.$$

The figure of exponential decay (26a) represents the formula $y = 2^{-x}$.

We shall concentrate on the part of the graph to the right of 0 on the x-axis. Figure 26b illustrates the exponential decline in plasma remifentanil concentration after a rapid intravenous bolus injection. Mathematically, this is $y = y_0.2^{-t/4.3}$. The half-life, i.e. the time it takes for the starting value to decline to 50%, is 3 min (see below). Apart from **time**, there are **other factors** which determine the rate of exponential decline; these can be summed together as the **elimination rate constant** k. The elimination rate constant is an analogy of the growth rate constant in the exponential growth process. The formula for physiological processes then becomes

$$y = y_0.e^{-kt}$$

where y_0, is the starting value, e is the base of natural logarithms, k is the elimination rate constant and t is time. We shall return to this formula later.

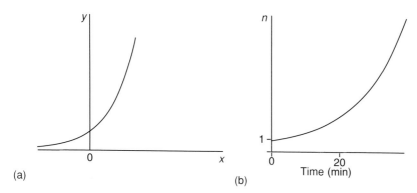

Figure 25. (a) Exponential growth curve. (b) growth of bacteria with time.

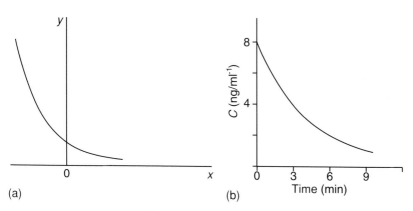

Figure 26. (a) Exponential decay curve. (b) exponential decline plasma remifentanil concentration.

Saturation exponential (e.g. pumping up a tyre, or intermittent positive pressure ventilation with a ventilator that generates constant pressure)

The process is reverse of exponential decay, but this time inverted around the x-axis, and it works against a limiting value. The formula therefore is

$$y = a - b^{-x},$$

where a is the limiting value, and the minus sign denotes the change in orientation around the x-axis (Figure 27a). A pure mathematical conversion of exponential decay would have no limiting value ($y = -b^{-x}$). The curve is symmetrical with the exponential growth curve across the zero point. Lung filling during intermittent positive pressure ventilation is depicted in Figure 27b. The exponential coefficient for lung filling is influenced by lung compliance and airway resistance. The larger either of these factors, the slower the lung filling, and conversely the smaller they are, the faster the lung filling. Thus the 'filling rate constant' is the inverse value of the product of lung compliance and airway resistance ($1/C.R$); their product, the reciprocal of the filling rate constant ($C.R$) is the time constant of the process (see below). Figure 27b represents the formula

$$Y = 500 - (500.e^{-t/300}).$$

The exponential formula is for convenience multiplied by the limiting value to obtain 0 for y at the beginning. The negative exponential factor $-1/300$ in the formula indicates that lung filling has a time constant of 300 ms.

Logarithm

Logarithm is the exponent to the power of which the base has to be raised to get the specified number. This complicated definition means that this is the reverse of exponential growth function (just as square root is the reverse of square function). Figure 28 resembles superficially saturation exponential, but it is different. The logarithmic curve is symmetrical with the exponential growth curve around the 45° axis, and it asymptotically approaches (never reaches) the y-axis: a logarithm of zero or negative numbers cannot be obtained, if the base (10 or e) is a positive number. y has no limit, which means it reaches infinity in both directions.

By contrast, a saturation exponential is symmetrical with the exponential decay curve around the x-axis; it asymptotically approaches the horizontal axis, or a limiting value above it, i.e. y has an upper limit.

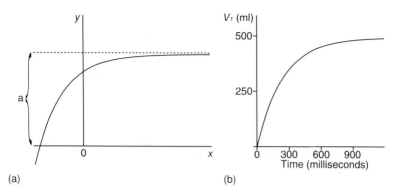

Figure 27. (a) Saturation exponential curve, (b) lung filling with a constant pressure generator.

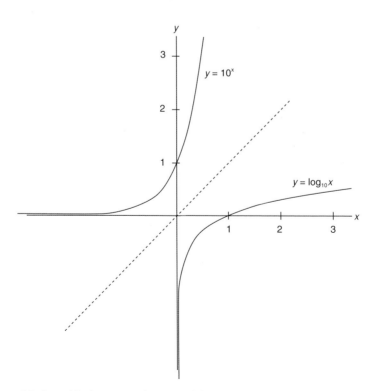

Figure 28. Logarithmic curve and exponential growth curve.

The exponential and logarithmic curves can be transformed into lines by plotting the values against a logarithmic scale. This scale has different properties from the usual linear scale: there is no zero (an exponential can never be zero), and the marks on the axis are equidistant for powers of the base. For instance, in the graph of $[H^+]$–pH relationship (see the chapter on pH measurement), notice that the logarithmic scale does not have zero and the distances between 1 and 10, and 10 and 100, are the same. The linear transformation of the curve is shown in that graph. The logarithmic scale is used in pharmacokinetics for linear transformation of elimination curves (see the chapter on pharmacokinetics).

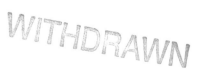

Exponentials 2: Properties of exponential decay curve

1. Decrease in constant proportion: in practice this means that the **rate of decrease depends on the 'mass' present**. The mass present at any point is graphically represented by the value of the ordinate (y-axis). The rate of decay is not constant, it is the **proportion** of the **mass that is 'lost'** that is **constant**: the previously introduced **elimination rate constant** in fact determines this fixed proportion eliminated per unit of time. For example, when emptying a bath across a fixed resistance (pipe), the flow rate (of emptying) depends directly on the hydrostatic pressure (the level of water) that changes as the bath empties, while the diameter of the pipe determines the proportion of contents that is emptied per unit of time, i.e. the elimination rate constant.

2. Every section of the curve differs from any other section by scale only: this follows from the first point: because the units of the y-axis are different from those of the x-axis (the time axis), the scale of the y-axis can be arbitrarily chosen. By the same token, any point of an exponential decay curve can be chosen as a 'starting point', and the vertical scale can be expanded if values are very small. In practice, this also means that we can project back and forward if we know a part of the curve.

3. The slope (tangent) at any point is directly proportional to y (the ordinate): this is also another way of saying the first point (the slope of the curve **is** the rate of decrease).

4. The vertical projection of the slope of the curve on the x-axis is constant. Properties 1, 2 and 4 are shown in Figure 29. Because the x-axis in natural processes represents time, τ is called the **time constant**. The time constant was already mentioned as the reciprocal value of the elimination rate constant. Therefore, this point is also indirectly connected with the first point: if we say a constant proportion per unit of time is lost, then the **time it takes to lose this proportion must be constant**. Think of the time constant as the **time to finish had the rate of decay been maintained**. This relationship holds no matter which starting value of y is chosen. In the bath analogy, the elimination rate constant is given by the resistance of the effluent pipe. This resistance is fixed for a given bath and can only let a certain flow of water through for a particular pressure. It follows that if the flow through the pipe were constant (i.e. driving pressure was constant), it would take a certain amount of time to pass a given volume of water: this time would be equal to the time constant of emptying by hydrostatic pressure. For different baths, the higher the resistance the smaller the flow for any given pressure, and the longer the emptying. In other words, the **elimination rate constant** (pipe resistance) and the **time constant** (time to empty if initial flow rate were maintained) are reciprocally related ($\tau = 1/k$), as said above. The exponential decay equation can then be written as:

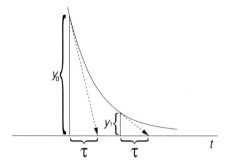

Figure 29. Rate of decay as a function of the ordinate, time constant as a projection of the tangent to the curve on the *x*-axis.

$y = y_0.e^{-kt}$ or $y = y_0.e^{-t/\tau}$. number e is the base of natural logarithms (= 2.718) and it has some unique properties, e.g. $de^t/dt = e^t$ (i.e. the rate of change of e^t with time has the same value as e^t). Returning to the bath analogy, this mathematical property means that volume or flow (the derivative of volume) can be charted on the ordinate, and the exponential decay curve will be identical. Any number can be chosen for the base constant, with appropriate adjustment of the scale; e was chosen because, as shown above, differentiation (and therefore integration) are very easy. Integration, or the area under the curve, is dealt with below.

5. **Area under the curve**: from any point to the infinitely remote point on the x-axis where the process may be thought of as having finished is **proportional to the ordinate** and it **is the product of the two fundamental determinants**, initial mass and time constant (y_0 and τ). In Figure 30, this is equal to the area of rectangle YOTY'. Calculation of the area under a curve is mathematically known as integration (see the chapter on flow). Thus, an operation that looks complicated (integration) is in fact very simple: $_0\int^\infty y_0.e^{-t/\tau}/dt = y_0.\tau$. Integration (for instance in the bath analogy) can be thought of as the summation of flow over time to measure volume. For a constant flow equal to the initial flow rate Q_0, the entire volume (area under the top horizontal line) would have taken τ time to disappear: that is the area of rectangle YOTY'. For the exponentially decreasing flow rate the process takes in theory infinity, but the total volume, the area under the exponential curve, in the end is the same.

Half-life, time constant and 'time to finish'

In pharmacology, half-life is used more than the time constant. It is the time taken for the mass to decrease to 50%. τ and half-life (t_{50}) are related and the latter is another type of time constant, but one with a more complicated relationship to the elimination rate constant than τ.

The percentage of mass left after a given time can be calculated for any exponential decay process. At time τ, the amount is:

$$y_\tau = y_0.e^{-\tau/\tau} = y_0.e^{-1} = y_0.0.37,$$

i.e. just over one-third of the initial amount. It follows that τ must be longer than the half-life because the proportion that is left is smaller. By substituting $y_0/2$ for y we find that τ is 1.44 times higher than the half-life.

Although in theory the process takes infinity, in practice we need to know how long it takes to complete. After a time equal to three time constants, y will be $y_0.e^{-3}$, or 5% of the initial value. After four time constants, y will be $y_0.e^{-4}$, or about 1% of the initial value. In other words, after four time constants the exponential decay process is for all intents and purposes finished.

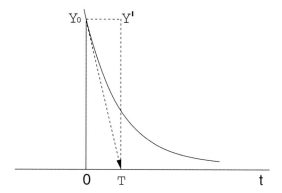

Figure 30. Area under the exponential curve equals the area of rectangle $Y_0 0 T Y'$.

Descriptive statistics

The purpose of statistical analysis is to obtain information from a **sample** that can then be extrapolated to a whole **population**; to analyse a whole population would be very lengthy, expensive and difficult to achieve. Care must be taken that the sample has the same characteristics as the target population (e.g. paediatric data cannot be extrapolated to the adult population).

Descriptive statistics categorise and summarise data. This chapter deals with summarisation of parametric (numerical) data.

To describe a population, or a sample, we should know its mode of distribution, a central point and its variability.

Variability is given by range, or by deviation from average. Only standard deviation is illustrated (but not derived) in this text.

Mode of distribution

Normal (Gaussian) distribution

This is the most frequent mode of distribution. The measured variable tends to cluster around the central, most common value, while extreme values either side of the centre are rare (e.g. adult male height, adult male haemoglobin). It is a bell-shaped curve only if the measurement was conducted in the whole population (e.g. the UK). Figure 31 shows the distribution of height in adult men. Observed values of height are plotted on the x-axis, and the frequency of observation (f) of each value is plotted against the y-axis. SD and $\bar{x}$ in the graph stand for standard deviation (SD) and mean (see below). 68% of population values lie within 1 SD from the population mean; 95.44% lie within 2 SD; and 95% lie within 1.96 SD. When studying a sample, the resulting frequency histogram (see the chapter on data presentation) would be less regular than the classic bell shape. Nevertheless, if the outline of a frequency histogram (Figure 32) approximates the bell shape, Gaussian distribution is assumed with all its characteristics.

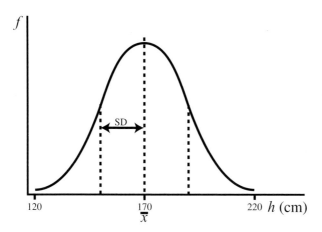

Figure 31. Normal distribution of height in adult men.

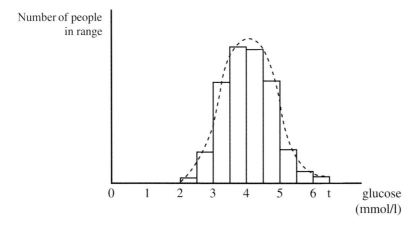

Figure 32. Gaussian distribution – blood glucose measurements in a large normal sample.

Log-normal or skewed distribution
This finding is fairly common in biological processes; the distribution can be converted to 'normal', i.e. Gaussian, by substituting natural logarithms for the observed values. For example, the distribution of hydrogen ion concentration in a normal population will be heavily skewed towards higher values, as the body tends towards acidosis. The most frequent value, 40 nmol/l, is lower than the arithmetic mean of the measured values (Figure 33).

Values < 20 are extremely rare, while those between 40 and 100 are rather common. A skew towards higher values is called a **positive skew**: the most frequent value is lower than the other measures of central tendency.

By converting hydrogen ion concentration to pH, the skew can be eliminated and the distribution will then be symmetrical around the central and most common value of 7.4, with the usual range narrowly clustered around this value.

An example of a **negative skew** is haemoglobin in women of reproductive age, where anaemia is fairly common: the most frequent value is higher than the other measures of central tendency (see Figure 34).

Other types of distribution
1. **Bimodal distribution** has two most common values, and thus gives the double hump appearance (Figure 35). Often a more detailed analysis reveals that, in fact, there are two different populations.
2. **J-shaped** distribution resembles a rising exponential process.
3. **U-shaped** distribution (e.g. cardiovascular mortality in relation to alcohol consumption) could perhaps be an 'inverse normal' distribution: if the curve was redrawn with 'survival rate' rather than mortality rate as the y-axis parameter, it would then resemble normal distribution with a central value between two and three units of alcohol.

Measures of central tendency

Mean $(\bar{x})$: $\bar{x} = \Sigma(x_i)/n$
The arithmetic mean, or average, is a common measure of central tendency. In a population normally distributed this is the value which is also the most frequent (mode), and which stands at midpoint (median) – see below. The process of summation is expressed as Σ.

Median
This is the 'middle' value, above and below which we find the values of 50% each for the rest of the population. In a positively skewed distribution the median will be higher than the most frequent value, but less than the arithmetic mean; the reverse applies in a negatively skewed distribution.

Mode
The mode is the most frequent value. In a skewed distribution it will be the *x*-axis value at the peak of the curve (note: not the peak value!). Bimodal distribution, as its name suggests, has two modes, i.e. two most frequent values.

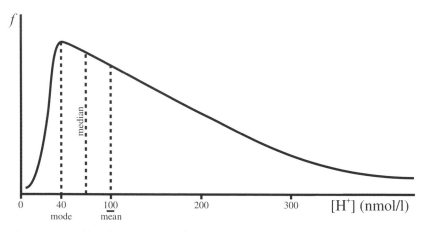

Figure 33. Positive skew – distribution of hydrogen ion concentration in humans.

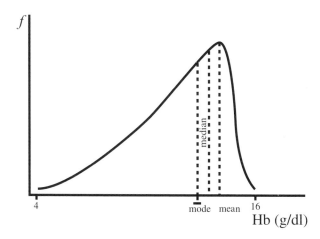

Figure 34. Negative skew – distribution of haemoglobin concentration in women.

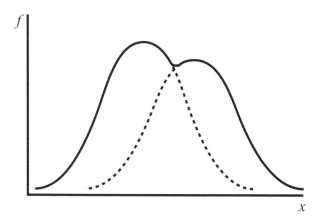

Figure 35. Bimodal distribution.

1 Presentation of data

The chapter on mathematical concepts deals with graphs as illustrations of relationships between variables. The chapter on descriptive statistics introduces statistical terms.

Diagrams

Diagrams are used to illustrate statistical data (see the chapter on descriptive statistics for explanation of terms).

The **pie diagram** is the simplest form. It is often used to illustrate data collected from audit. It is useful if there are several categories (portions) of a whole, for instance age groups, different surgical specialties, items of expenditure in budget, etc. The pie diagram gives an immediate idea of how the whole is divided up. Figure 36 shows all patients who experienced nausea after surgery according to the type of operation.

The **histogram** is best used to show counts – integer numbers of patients, objects or days. Bands or columns are used for the illustration; although each number has only one dimension, plotted against the y-axis, the second dimension – the width of the band – makes the visual distinction between groups easier and distinguishes a histogram from a line graph. Figure 37 shows the comparison of the incidence of postoperative nausea among men and women. Measurements of continuously variable data are best represented by scatter diagram (see below) although the histogram is often used in this situation.

The **frequency histogram** illustrates the **distribution** of different values of a measured variable in a certain sample or population. Figure 38 shows the distribution of hypothetical laboratory measurements of fasting blood glucose concentration in all employees of a hospital. The x-axis is divided into bands of integer numbers of blood glucose measurements; the height of each band represents the number of people with this value. Notice that the histogram is used correctly in this situation: integer numbers of people are plotted on the y-axis. If the number in each group is expressed as a percentage of the total, this histogram becomes the frequency histogram. For a normal sample the outline of the frequency histogram will resemble the bell-shape of Gaussian distribution (see the chapter on descriptive statistics).

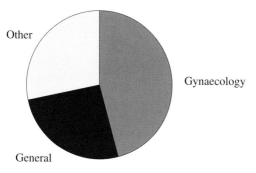

Figure 36. Pie diagram – proportion of nausea and vomiting according to the type of surgery in a large sample of day surgical patients.

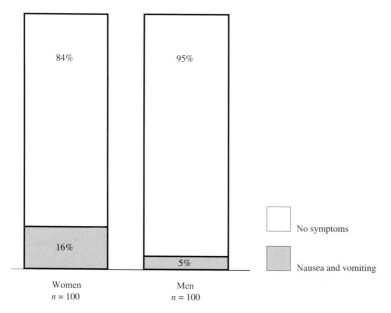

Figure 37. Histogram (bar diagram) – incidence of postoperative nausea and vomiting in men and women after day surgery procedures.

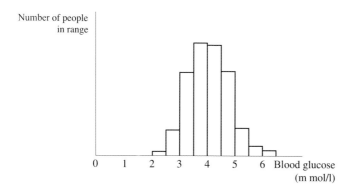

Figure 38. Frequency histogram.

Scatter diagrams or line drawings should be used for plotting results of measurements; for few measurements, each result is plotted as a point defined by its coordinates. If a trend is observed, this is represented by the line of best fit, or **regression line**. Individual measurements should lie close to this line. The measure of this closeness is called the **correlation coefficient**. For a perfect fit the correlation coefficient is 1 or –1 (Figure 39); when there is no agreement between the points and regression line, the correlation coefficient is 0 (Figure 40). Care must be taken to include sufficient number of valid data: an isolated outlier in a small sample of otherwise random values probably means that the measurement was incorrect or that the individual comes from a different population.

For a large number of measurements each point in the graph represents the central value, usually the mean, and error bars should be included to indicate the dispersion of each group. The points are usually joined by lines to show any trend – **line drawing**. Figure 41 shows mean pain scores in a group of 20 surgical patients on intramuscular 'as required' analgesia, and 20 surgical patients on patient-controlled analgesia. Error bars overlap immediately after the operation but there seems a trend for improved pain relief with patient-controlled analgesia.

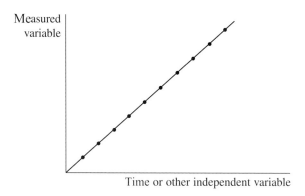

Figure 39. Correlation coefficient = 1.

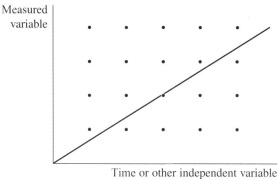

Figure 40. Correlation coefficient = 0.

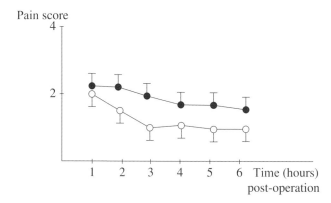

Figure 41. Line drawing with error bars – average pain scores after total abdominal hysterectomy in patients on morphine patient controlled analgesia (o) and on intramuscular morphine on demand (•).

Receiver operating characteristic curve

Sensitivity (detection of true positives) and **specificity** (detection of true negatives) of a test are important properties. In an ideal case each should be **equal to 100%** or the value of 1.0: all true positives should be identified by a test and all true negatives rejected, or fall below a cut-off value. In practice, this is rarely the case. A **trade-off** usually has to be sought between a good enough sensitivity and an acceptable specificity.

The name 'receiver operating characteristic' (ROC) curves was conceived during the Second World War to name the ability of radar operators to discriminate between friend or enemy blips on the screen, whilst also discounting the background noise (false positives). When tested, correct or false answers could be plotted and the result was the ROC curve. This was later taken up by the medical profession to describe the accuracy of laboratory tests.

To visualize how **false positives and false negatives are related** to the true values and to each other, consider Figure 42. It shows the distribution of fasting blood sugar in the normal (non-diabetic) population and in the diabetic population. Note that the distribution curve for diabetics is skewed to the right. Some overlap exists between the two populations, as not all diabetics will always have a raised fasting blood sugar, whilst a raised fasting blood sugar may on occasions be seen in a non-diabetic person.

The area where the two curves **overlap** is shown in grey. It is a roughly triangular area with a peak at point A (the cut-off blood sugar level of 5.5 mmol l^{-1}). To the left of the separation point in this **grey area** lie the **false negative** (diabetics classified as 'normal'), and to the right the **false positives** (non-diabetics diagnosed as diabetics).

If we artificially move **the cut-off point** for 'normal' **to the left**, say point B (peak of the distribution curve for non-diabetics), we would **increase** the number of **false positives** while at the same time the false negative rate would decrease. Diabetes would be wrongly diagnosed in a higher proportion of normal population but very few true diabetics would be missed. The reverse would happen if the cut-off point was moved to the right, to a higher level of fasting blood sugar (point C).

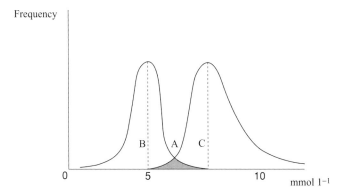

Figure 42. Frequency distribution of tasting blood sugar in normal and diabetic population.

Figure 43 plots ROC curves, as described above, for various tests. **Sensitivity** (true positive rate) is plotted on the *y*-axis against (**1 - specificity**) – true negative rate on the *x*-axis. Looking at Figure 1, it is obvious that if there was **no overlap** between the two populations tested, the distribution curves would be completely separated. There would be **no false positives** and **no false negatives** if the cut off point was placed correctly. Testing such ideal populations with this cut-off point would show a sensitivity and specificity of 1.0. By artificially moving the cut-off point to lie within one or the other population, we would allow either false positives (by moving to the left towards point B) or false negatives (by moving to the right towards point C). The ROC plot of this ideal situation is shown in Figure 43 as a thick black line and is formed by the *y*-axis and its coordinate at the value of 1.0. The area under this curve is equal to 1.0 (it is a square equal to the area of the graph).

In real life, as shown in Figure 42, overlap exists and therefore false positives and false negatives co-exist. For most tests, it makes sense to put the cut-off point at point A – the mid-point between the peaks of the distribution curves, i.e. where both specificity and sensitivity are highest. A test which discriminates well between the two populations tested produces a **good ROC curve**. This is shown as a thin black line, and it will **approximate the ideal** described above. The area under the curve will approximate 1.0. In this case, the test discriminates well between the two populations, and such test would be a gold standard.

In some circumstances, it may be better to **increase sensitivity at the expense of specificity** or vice versa. One such case is prediction of the difficult airway. It is desirable that every difficult airway is identified as such (sensitivity of 100%). Because of overlap of 'normal' and 'difficult', and because the cut-off point is moved into the 'normal' area (analogous to point B in Figure 42), one has to accept a high number of false positives – normal airway identified as difficult. In practice no single test fulfils even this criterion and we have to apply a battery of tests to improve the results.

Figure 43 also shows a straight interrupted line, the diagonal of the area of the plot. This represents an imaginary test which does not discriminate between the two popluations tested, i.e. a useless or irrelevant test. Identification of true positives and true negatives in this case is purely by chance. The area under this line is equal to 0.5 (half of the square). The more a ROC curve approximates this line, and the area under it 0.5, the less useful the test.

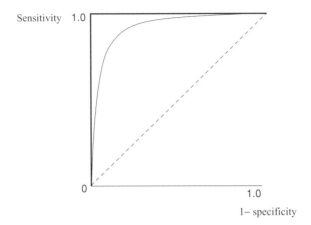

Figure 43. ROC curves.

Gas supply and pressure

Medical gases supplied in cylinders are compressed to a high pressure in order to store a big mass in a relatively small volume (it follows from Boyle's law that the higher the pressure inside the cylinder, the bigger the final volume of decompressed gas). The human respiratory system operates at low pressures; high pressure can produce barotrauma. Gas supply pressure has to be reduced in stages and safety features are incorporated. The wide range of pressures in the medical gas supply and in the breathing system has led to the establishment of various units suiting each particular purpose: bars for high pressures, lb/psi for moderate pressures, mmHg for atmospheric and lower pressures, and cmH_2O for very low pressures measured as a column of water. (See more on gas pressure in the chapter on real gas compression, and on units in simple mechanics.)

Figure 44 shows the pressures inside the gas supply system on a logarithmic scale; in this way, it is possible to include a wide range of pressures in one graph. In particular, notice that the gas supply operates in terms of hundreds of kPa (bars) but the breathing system pressures are kPa units or their fractions. The logarithmic scale of the ordinate also demonstrates that each stage of decompression reduces the pressure very approximately by a factor of 10.

The volume shown on the abscissa is that which would be obtained by decompression of 1 litre gas at the pressure indicated to atmospheric pressure. This volume can be calculated by using the formula

$$V = p_c + p_a = p_c + 1$$

for 1 litre gas decompressed to 1 atmosphere, where p_c = cylinder pressure.

Pressure conversion

$1 \, atm = 101.3 \, kPa = 760 \, mmHg = 1033 \, cmH_2O = 14.69 \, lb/in^2$
$100 \, kPa = 1 \, bar$. Notice that $1000 \, kPa = 1 \, MPa$ (megapascal) $= 10 \, bar$, and, by approximation, $1 \, kPa = 10 \, cmH_2O = 7.5 \, mm \, Hg$.

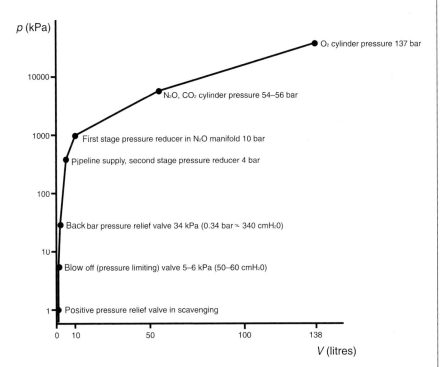

Figure 44. Pressure/volume relationship in medical gas supply.

The circle system is a semiclosed or closed absorption system; with the absorber out of circuit it becomes a semiclosed rebreathing system. Low flow can be used because carbon dioxide (CO_2) is absorbed and this gives economy of use and produces little pollution. Low flow has been defined as a total fresh gas flow of 1 l/minute, and minimum flow as 0.5 l/minute. Most new anaesthetic machines incorporate a circle system with absorber, unidirectional valves and exhaust valve removed from the patient end (see Figure 45). Modern highly efficient vaporizers are situated outside the circuit.

The most common **technical problem** with the circle system **is disconnection of fresh gas** flow at the fresh gas flow outlet and **shutting off the expiratory valve** when the intended mode of ventilation is spontaneous breathing (by leaving the control knob turned to 'ventilator' instead of 'bag').

Performance of the circle system under low fresh gas flow conditions

Inspired gas composition will be identical to the fresh gas composition at high fresh gas flows, as the expired gas will be flushed out of the system, and CO_2 is absorbed. When reducing the gas flow to low levels, the expired gas will make an increasingly bigger contribution to the gas composition inside the circuit. Oxygen flow must not be reduced below the minimum 250 ml/min, the basic metabolic requirement being 200 ml/min. The **concentration effect** will influence the inspired gas composition at induction, when anaesthetic (nitrous oxide, or N_2O) uptake is high. Alveolar oxygen concentration will increase, and N_2O concentration will decrease; if very low gas flows were used during induction, alveolar N_2O concentration could be below MAC. Therefore, it is necessary to maintain a high fresh gas flow during induction and until expired concentration of the anaesthetic is near inspired concentration (about 10 min). After this, anaesthetic uptake is low, and thus alveolar concentration of the anaesthetic rises, while alveolar pO_2 decreases. Such hypothetical situations are illustrated in Figure 46: 50% O_2 and N_2O are supplied in a circle system, with assumptions about O_2 consumption, CO_2 production and absorption. At fresh gas flows > 2 litres, inspired gas composition closely approximates the fresh gas composition, regardless of uptake. At lower flows, nitrous oxide uptake plays an increasingly important role: when nitrous oxide uptake is high, alveolar oxygen concentration rises steeply (the concentration effect is more pronounced) but when the uptake decreases to < 200 ml/min, alveolar oxygen concentration decreases substantially < 50%, as nitrous oxide is then taken up at a lower rate than oxygen.

The inspired concentration of anaesthetic vapour is affected by its own uptake; therefore, when uptake is high the inspired concentration of the vapour will decrease and vice versa.

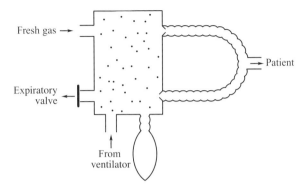

Figure 45. The circle system.

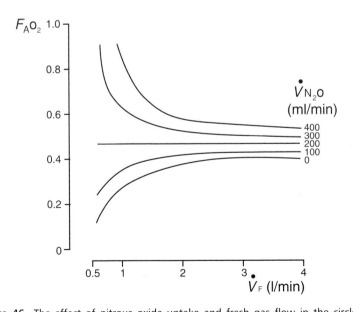

Figure 46. The effect of nitrous oxide uptake and fresh gas flow in the circle system on alveolar oxygen concentration. Reproduced with permission from Butterworth-Heinemann.

Another factor affecting the inspired gas composition is the accompanying steady washout of nitrogen from the body. One litre of nitrogen contained in the lungs is washed out during the induction with high gas flow. Thereafter, nitrogen accumulates in the circuit at very low flows, further lowering the inspired pO_2. The volatile agent concentration is also lowered by the accumulated nitrogen, and this tends to offset the expected rise in inspired vapour concentration when vapour uptake is low.

Uptake of inhalational agents is an exponential decay process, and accumulation of nitrogen in the circuit a saturation exponential. Both processes have a **time constant** τ, that is directly proportional to the volume of the system V, and inversely proportional to the difference between fresh gas flow and the sum of all gas uptake. Thus, in theory if the fresh gas flow exactly equalled all gas uptake, the time constant would be infinitely high (because then $\tau = V/0$). With fresh gas flows being somewhat (e.g. 10%) above the basal requirement, the time constant would still be several hours, offering a protection from a dangerous mixture being delivered. At the other end of the spectrum, with fresh gas flow much in excess of anaesthetic uptake the time constant is short but at these high flow rates anaesthetic uptake and nitrogen washout do not affect the inspired gas composition.

At minimal flow, the anaesthetist must also consider if a sufficient **amount (mass) of vapour** is being delivered. In practice, this could happen with enflurane which has a relatively high MAC and a higher blood/gas solubility than isoflurane. Its uptake is therefore much higher than that of halothane or isoflurane. Figure 47 illustrates the uptake of the three inhalational agents during anaesthesia in a patient weighing 90 kg when the inspired concentration of the agent is set so that the expired concentration is around 0.8 MAC. The uptake of isoflurane after 10 minutes is less than 30 ml/minute but uptake of enflurane is still nearly 60 ml/minute. Assuming that after 10 minutes fresh gas flow is reduced to 0.5 l/minute with the highest vaporizer setting (5%), the system will only deliver 25 ml of vapour every minute (5% of 0.5 l is 25 ml). The inspired concentration of isoflurane can thus just about keep up with its continued uptake but if enflurane is used the system is unable to deliver sufficient vapour at this minimal flow; flow reduction can only be effected when uptake has decreased near the maximum vaporizer output at minimal flow. In leaner patients, this can be done after some 15 to 20 minutes. Alternatively, a higher inspired concentration could be used from the start (e.g. to obtain expired concentration 1.2 MAC, to accelerate the initial high uptake period) or flow could be reduced in stages. At one litre per minute, vaporizer output at 5% is 50 ml and would cover enflurane uptake after 15 minutes even in the oversize patient.

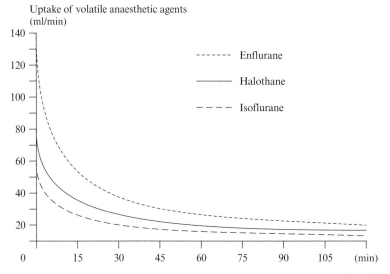

Uptake of volatile anaesthetic agents, desired expiratory concentration value: $0.8 \times$ MAC

Figure 47. Uptake of volatile anaesthetic as a function of time. Reproduced with permission from Butterworth-Heinemann.

The Mapleson A (Magill) breathing system

Conway (1985) described the geometry of the Mapleson classification and the behaviour of the breathing systems under conditions of spontaneous and controlled respiration. The Mapleson A (Magill) system (Figure 48) has the fresh gas inlet remote from the subject while the expiratory valve is near the subject. Dead space is shown as the shaded area. This makes the system particularly **economic to use during spontaneous respiration**.

Figure 49 shows the hypothetical pressure and flow inside the Mapleson A system during expiration. Flow during expiration, which is usually a passive process, is maximal at the beginning of expiration, and it falls off exponentially. Pressure inside the system rises exponentially but at a faster rate than the expiratory flow falls because of accumulation of fresh gas in the system; this rise in pressure is cut off when the expiratory valve opens at 5–6 kPa and this pressure is then maintained until end-expiration. Areas under the flow curve give expired volumes (see the chapter on flow and volume measurement); dead space gas (V_D), which is identical in composition to fresh gas is expired first until point A on the graph. When the expiratory valve opens at point B, alveolar gas (V_A) beyond that point is vented out. Furthermore, alveolar gas that was deposited inside the system between points A and B (start of alveolar gas expiration and opening of expiratory valve) is after the opening of expiratory valve being pushed out by the fresh gas inflow (V_F). If sufficient time is allowed after the opening of the expiratory valve to allow venting of the alveolar gas deposited during the valve closure, at end-expiration the system will only contain fresh gas and dead space gas (identical in composition). Thus, during spontaneous respiration, provided that **fresh gas flow is at least equal to alveolar ventilation**, i.e. about 70% of the minute volume, there will be no rebreathing of CO_2-containing gas. During **controlled ventilation** the **economy of gas flow is lost**: positive pressure is applied during inspiration and the pressure relief valve therefore opens, venting fresh gas; furthermore, the valve needs to be set to a higher pressure (tightened) and therefore during expiration it opens later, allowing retention of CO_2-containing gas inside the system. Higher flows are, therefore, needed during controlled ventilation. This disadvantage of the Magill system, and the large weight of the expiratory valve and scavenging close to the subject (i.e. to the mask or airway connection), caused a steady decline in the popularity of the Magill system. It is being increasingly replaced by the T-piece or circle absorption system.

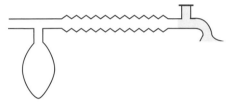

Figure 48. The Mapleson A breathing system.

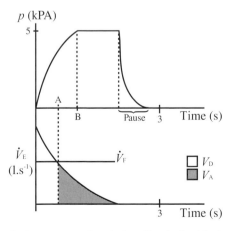

Figure 49. Hypothetical pressure and expiratory flow in the Mapleson A system.

T-pieces

T-pieces (Figure 50) are geometrically opposite of the Magill system: the fresh gas flow inlet is near the subject while the expiratory valve or port is the furthest. E type is a valveless system suitable for spontaneously breathing subjects only. F type is a paediatric valveless system.

Figure 51 shows theoretical inspiratory gas flow during **spontaneous breathing** in a T-piece system. The inspiratory waveform is a sine wave. Integration of flow (area under the curve) yields volume inspired. This is again divided into gas that enters alveoli (V_A) and dead space gas (V_D). Superimposed on the graph is the fresh gas flow, which is constant. The area under the straight line of the fresh gas flow is the fresh gas volume delivered into the system. It can be seen that at point A the inspiratory flow exceeds the fresh gas flow. Until that point, excess fresh gas was being deposited in the tubing. After that point, inspiratory flow is supplied in part (the part exceeding fresh gas flow) by gas previously deposited in the tubing. Provided that the roughly triangular area between the fresh gas flow line, the inspiratory curve up to point A, and the y-axis, which is the **volume deposited in the large bore tubing**, **equals** the area under the peak inspiratory flow above the fresh gas flow line up to point B (which is the **volume of gas drawn from the system in excess of fresh gas flow** during that time), no CO_2-containing gas will be rebreathed. These conditions will apply if **fresh gas flow** is approximately **twice the minute volume** during **spontaneous respiration**.

During **controlled ventilation**, fresh gas flow mixes with expired gas as the peak ventilatory flows are higher; the inspirate will then contain CO_2. Under these conditions the magnitude of rebreathing will depend on fresh gas flow and minute ventilation: an increase in either of these will lower arterial CO_2 tension. In fact, arterial partial pressure of CO_2 becomes the product of fresh gas flow and minute ventilation. To maintain the CO_2 level, an inverse relationship must be maintained between fresh gas flow and minute volume. If **minute ventilation is increased**, **fresh gas flow can be reduced**; this provides economy of flow **during controlled ventilation**.

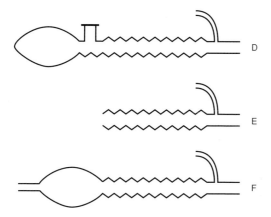

Figure 50. T-pieces.

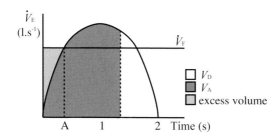

Figure 51. Inspiratory flow and fresh gas flow in the Bain system. Reproduced with permission from Butterworth-Heinemann.

Lung filling with automatic lung ventilators

Constant pressure generator

This type of ventilator is driven by fresh gas flow (Manley) or by electricity (East Radcliffe). It is suitable for lungs with relatively normal characteristics because the generated pressure is relatively low (25–30 cmH$_2$O). When a step change in pressure is generated, the difference (Δp) between pressure at the mouth (p$_m$) and alveolar pressure (p$_A$) results in gas flow. As the lungs are being filled by the gas, this pressure difference falls in an exponential fashion, and so does flow. The lung filling curve (volume–time–relationship) is a saturation exponential. The time constant of the lung filling process is the product of lung compliance C and airways resistance R ($\tau = C.R$): see the chapter on exponentials. Figure 52a shows the filling of a normal lung, the pressures, flow and volume are plotted against the time. P_A denotes alveolar pressure; P_M pressure at the mouth; V = gas flow and V = volume achieved. For a high airways resistance (Figure 52b) the time constant is long: the filling takes longer. This is because the high airways resistance reduces the flow from the beginning ($V = \Delta p/R$). For a poorly compliant lung (Figure 52c), the time constant is shortened. The flow initially is unaltered but it decreases quickly as the stiff lung soon opposes further filling. Thus the final volume achieved is reduced.

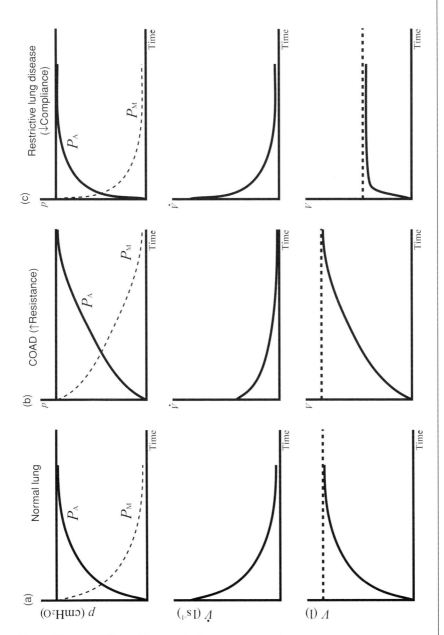

Figure 52. Lung filling with a constant pressure generator.

Constant flow generator

This type of ventilator is suitable for **lungs with abnormal characteristics**. It can generate constant flow by passing gas driven by high pressure through a flow restrictor. High-pressure gas can be the sole driving force (Penlon) or sophisticated electronic circuitry generates the pressures and flows required (Ohmeda 7900, or most ventilators suitable for intensive therapy). Figure 53 again shows lung filling for a normal lung, a lung with a high airway resistance and a poorly compliant lung. The sequence of graphs is altered to progress from the flow generated, through volume delivered to pressures achieved.

Constant flow generated by the ventilator is reflected in a constant volume delivered in a chosen time, as volume is the integral of flow. Thus the flow and volume graphs are the same for all three situations. From experience, it is known that pressures achieved will depend on lung characteristics. As the normal lungs are filled (first column), alveolar pressure, p_A, rises in line with lung volume. Alveolar pressure can be calculated as the ratio of lung volume delivered and lung compliance (as lung compliance is the ratio of lung volume over alveolar pressure: $C = V/p_A$). Pressure difference between alveolar pressure and pressure at the mouth is given as the product of flow (which is constant) and resistance ($\Delta p = V.R$), and is therefore constant. Pressure at the mouth is a simple sum of alveolar pressure and the pressure difference ($p_m = \dot{V}/C + \dot{V}.R$).

For a high airway resistance (second column), the pressure difference between alveolar pressure and mouth pressure will be higher, as is obvious from the above formula. Pressure at the mouth, therefore, will reflect this higher pressure difference. The set lung volume will be delivered but at the expense of a higher pressure at the mouth.

For a poorly compliant lung (third column), alveolar pressure will rise more steeply as it will reach a higher value for a given lung volume (alveolar pressure and lung compliance are inversely related – see the formula above), and this will be reflected in a higher mouth pressure. A set lung volume will be delivered again at the expense of a higher pressure at the mouth.

To avoid barotrauma, pressure limits must be set on this type of ventilator; for very stiff lungs, pressure-controlled ventilation is used that keeps the driving pressure constant at a chosen setting. The price to pay is a smaller volume delivered, leading to CO_2 retention – permissive hypercapnia.

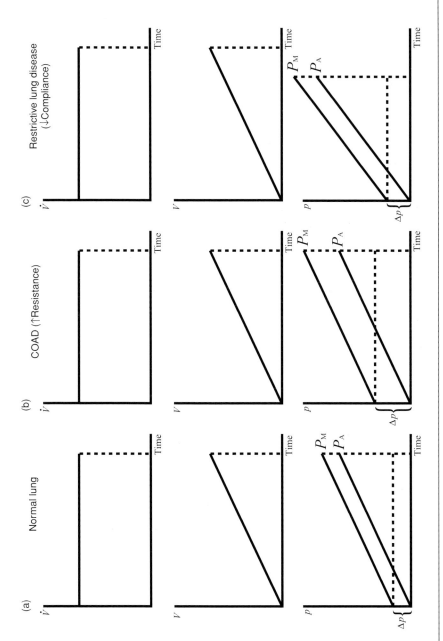

Figure 53. Lung filling with a constant flow generator.

Part 2

Clinical measurement

Basic measurement concepts

Physical and physiological variables are measured using an instrument that converts the measured quantity (the input signal) into an electrical (output) signal. The signal is then amplified, displayed and recorded in analogue (wave) or digital (numeric) form. Figures 54–56 illustrate some comparisons between the measured quantity (the 'true' value) represented by the black continuous line, and the output of an instrument, represented by the individual dots (measurements).

For accurate measurement, the system must fulfil the following criteria:

1. Static accuracy – this means that:

• The output signal is directly proportional to the input signal – the **linearity principle**. For linear relationship, see the chapter on mathematical concepts. Figure 54 shows test results of two new glucometers compared with a 'gold standard'. The first apparatus conforms to the linearity principle but deviates somewhat from the true value on either side: it is fairly accurate, but not precise. The second apparatus shows consistently lower results: it is precise but not accurate. The gold standard apparatus, of course, must be both precise and accurate.

• There is neither baseline nor sensitivity **drift**, i.e. the output signal does not deviate from true zero in time, with changes in temperature or other factors – see Figure 53.

• There is absence of **hysteresis**, i.e. that the system's response is identical whether the input signal is applied in an incremental or decremental manner. Systems exhibiting hysteresis thus produce a signal that forms **a loop** (see Figure 56); its rate of rise is slow at first and faster at higher values of upward increments. Conversely, when the input signal is decreasing, the output signal falls off slowly at first but the rate of decrease is faster near the lowest point. Such a loop resembles the compliance loop, and indeed the property of hysteresis can be thought of as the 'compliance' of the system.

2. Physiological reactance – this means that the measuring system does not affect the process being measured.

3. Dynamic accuracy – to fulfil this requirement, the system must faithfully record rapidly changing events. This means that the system must accurately reproduce both the amplitude of each harmonic component (see the chapter on mathematical concepts and sine wave), and their phase relationship.

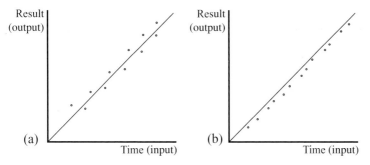

Figure 54. Linearity principle: (a) measurement accurate but impercise. (b) measurement precise but inaccurate.

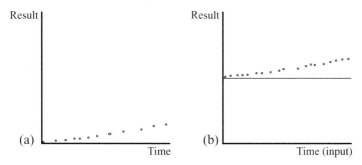

Figure 55. Drift: (a) baseline (zero) drift. (b) sensitivity drift.

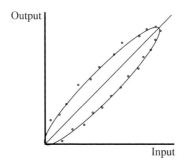

Figure 56. Hysteresis loop.

To avoid **amplitude distortion** the system must have a **frequency response** higher than the highest harmonic. For instance, at a heart rate of 120 beats min^{-1}, the frequency of an associated signal (e.g. blood pressure) is 2 Hz. Assuming that at least 10 harmonics are needed for an accurate reproduction of the input signal, the system's amplitude–frequency response must be about 20 Hz.

Phase distortion is frequency-dependent. **Critical damping** extinguishes natural oscillations of the system and abolishes phase distortion; all the harmonics will be recorded with the same time delay and the output signal will be undistorted although delayed in time. See the chapter on electromanometers and Figure 57 for more detail.

Noise, i.e. a false signal, will also reduce dynamic accuracy depending on its frequency. Static accuracy will not be affected as new machines can filter out background noise or disregard it. The stronger the input signal and the weaker the noise, i.e. the higher the **signal-to-noise ratio**, the better dynamic accuracy.

To satisfy the above criteria, **calibration** is required. This is achieved by the application of static increments and decrements of input signal and recording the response. Drift is established by leaving the system with the desired input signal for several hours.

The dynamic response is tested by a stepwise application of a large signal and its sudden removal, as illustrated opposite.

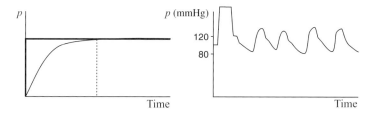

Figure 57. Critical damping ($\xi = 1$).

Electromanometers, frequency response and damping

An electromanometer is a device for direct (invasive) blood pressure measurement. The sensor is **a pressure transducer**, a device that converts mechanical energy to electrical signals: blood pressure oscillations are conducted along a fluid-filled tube (catheter) to a chamber that has a flexible diaphragm on the end (shown in Figure 58). Displacement of the diaphragm by these oscillations is sensed electrically and converted into an electrical signal.

Frequency response

After a single change in pressure inside the system, the fluid continues to move in oscillations as it is reflected from the diaphragm on one side and blood vessel wall on the other. The frequency of this oscillatory movement is inherent to the set-up and is called the **resonant** or natural undamped **frequency**, f_n.

To follow the measured pressure the system must be able to respond quickly: its frequency response must be higher than the highest frequency measured.

The frequency response (natural resonant frequency) is calculated using the formula:

$$f_n = r/2\sqrt{S/\pi\rho l}$$

It can be seen that a large-bore catheter (large radius r) of short length (l), a stiff diaphragm (S), plus fluid of low density (ρ), are the requirements for a high natural resonant frequency of an electromanometer.

Damping

For correct operation, the system has to be able to respond adequately to the highest frequency contained in the transducer waveform. Therefore, it has to respond quickly. However, a high natural resonant frequency of the system would produce natural oscillations at that frequency, which could interfere with the recorded frequency. Damping is the **tendency to extinguish natural oscillations** through viscous and frictional forces. In the mechanical model this is provided by immersing a spring in a viscous fluid, which slows down and extinguishes the natural oscillations. The same factors that influence natural frequency also influence damping but in an inverse manner; in addition, the viscous resistance, as known from the Hagen–Poiseuille formula, is directly proportional to viscosity, η. In the clinical situation, the specific fluid viscous resistance and density are constant and can be ignored. Dextrose is used because it is a non-ionic solution.

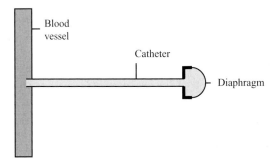

Figure 58. Electromanometer principle.

It follows from the above that the factors that we can use to manipulate the response of the system are **catheter length**, its **diameter** and diaphragm **stiffness**. Long and narrow catheters reduce the frequency response, and increase damping.

Figures 57 and 59–61 illustrate four situations with different degrees of damping.

1. In a system where damping is virtually absent ($\zeta \to 0$), a stepwise pressure change results in an overshoot followed by oscillations at natural frequency. Such a situation would arise if the catheter is relatively wide and short. In the corresponding arterial blood pressure trace, note the natural oscillations after a flush and on the trace, and overshoot of the signal.
2. At the other extreme, if a long and very narrow catheter is used, damping is greatly increased ($\zeta \gg 1$), and the system is unable to respond quickly to the pressure change. The graphic recording is that of a slow-rising saturation exponential curve. The corresponding blood pressure trace has a more rounded form with loss of detail; oscillations after flush are absent. In the extreme case, the pressure trace almost converges on the mean blood pressure.
3. If we manipulate the parameters in such a way that the system responds more quickly but just avoids overshooting, damping is said to be **critical** ($\zeta = 1$) (Figure 57). Natural oscillation after flush is absent in the hypothetical arterial blood pressure trace but some loss of detail is still present.
4. The situation above is clearly not the best solution, as the response of the system may not be fast enough to follow the higher frequencies. Therefore, damping is further reduced (catheter shorter and wider, diaphragm stiffer) to allow a small overshoot. Experimentally it was found that the best compromise between accuracy and speed is achieved when damping is two-thirds of critical ($\zeta = 0.66$): this is optimal damping (Figure 61). On the arterial blood pressure trace, the small overshoot is found as a single oscillation after flush, and it can be seen that detail is preserved without distortion by oscillations. A too damped trace on the pressure recording may be due to the presence of air, or to partial blockage of the catheter by clot, resolved by removal of air and by flushing of the line.

Another factor that can be accidentally or deliberately introduced is an air bubble: this interrupts the fluid column and in effect reduces the stiffness of the diaphragm, as air is compressible. The presence of air therefore reduces the frequency response of the system, and increases damping. See also the chapter on basic measurement concepts.

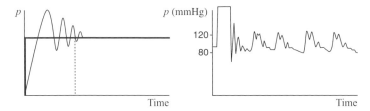

Figure 59. Low damping ($\xi \to 0$).

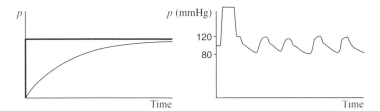

Figure 60. High damping ($\xi \gg 1$).

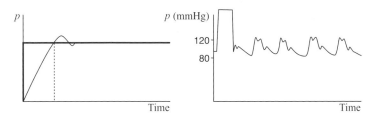

Figure 61. Optimal damping ($\xi = 0.66$).

Pulse oximeter principle

An oximeter is an instrument designed to measure oxygen saturation of haemoglobin in whole blood. Oxygen saturation (S_aO_2) is defined as the ratio of oxygen content of haemoglobin over oxygen carrying capacity.

Oximeters operate on the principle of light absorption; the formula below expresses the **Lambert–Beer law:**

$$I = I_o \cdot e^{-c.d.E},$$

where I, I_o = received and initial light intensity; c = concentration of absorbing medium; e = the base of natural logarithms; d = distance travelled; and E = the extinction coefficient of a particular medium.

The exponential coefficient has three components: E, which is fixed for each medium, c (concentration) and d (distance), which can be varied. Figure 62 shows light absorbances of oxyhaemoglobin, deoxyhaemoglobin, methaemoglobin and carboxyhaemoglobin, in the red and infra-red spectrum. It can be seen that the lines of oxy-and deoxyhaemoglobin cross several times, and deviate most widely at 660 nm wavelength. The points where these two lines cross indicate the wavelength at which the light absorbances are equal; such a point is called an **isobestic point**. The 800 nm point was used as a reference point to compensate for changes in total haemoglobin concentration (light absorbance at this point does not depend on oxyhaemoglobin concentration). The light absorbance of a given sample of blood at 660 nm (or any other point chosen) will lie somewhere between the two curves, depending on the percentage of oxyhaemoglobin concentration (c), which is in fact oxygen saturation.

Pulse oximeter components and method of measurement

The pulse oximeter consists of two light-emitting diodes, a photocell detector and a microprocessor with a visual display unit. The light-emitting diodes are illuminated in turn at a set frequency, and an off phase is incorporated to compensate for extraneous light. The wavelengths chosen in practice are actually 660 nm (red) and 940 nm (infrared), since this gives a better separation of the wavelengths (i.e. the newer machines do not utilize the isobestic point). At 940 nm the light absorbance of deoxyhaemoglobin is less than that of oxyhaemoglobin, while at 660 nm the absorbances are reversed. However, linear relationship of the light absorbances ratio to oxygen saturation still applies, as shown in Figure 63.

The detector cannot distinguish between different wavelengths, therefore it assumes that light received is that from the light-emitting diode currently on. Light absorption varies with cardiac cycle because of the difference in oxyhaemoglobin percentage between arterial and venous blood. This variation is detected at the two wavelengths, and pulse rate calculated.

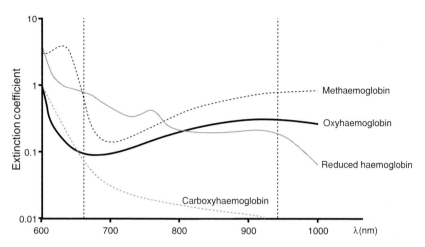

Figure 62. Pulse oximeter principle. Extinction coefficients of oxyhaemoglobin, reduced haemoblobin, ethaemoglobin and carboxyheamoblobin in red and infrared light.

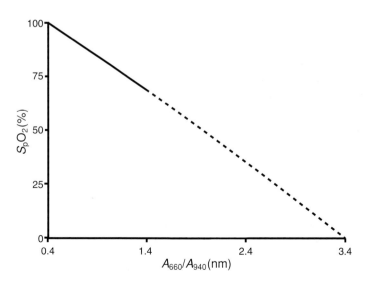

Figure 63. Relationship between saturation of arterial blood with oxygen and the light absorbances ratio of haemoglobin.

The pulse oximeter detects the cyclical change in light absorption in the arterial end of the capillaries as well as constant light absorption by venous blood and tissues. The constant absorption is ignored, and pulse waveform displayed based on the changing absorption by 'arterial' blood, as shown in Figure 64.

There are numerous sources of error and interference which include physiological and physical factors (vasoconstriction, hypotension, additional arterial or venous pulsations, scattering and refraction of light, time delay), intrinsic and extrinsic factors (other types of haemoglobin, dyes, nail varnish, patient movement, diathermy, ambient light). Inherent error is less than +/–3% at saturations > 70%.

Pulse oximetry as a form of monitoring has many advantages: it is a continuous non-invasive method of measurement of haemoglobin oxygen saturation, gives early warning of hypoxic events, and is superior to clinical judgement. Easy to use, with little interpretation needed, it is one of the minimum monitoring requirements. The main danger is a false sense of security when used to detect hypoxaemia at high inspired oxygen concentrations.

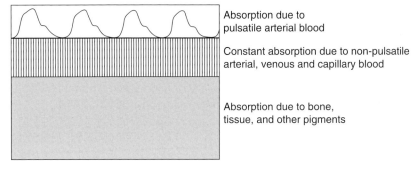

Absorption due to
pulsatile arterial blood

Constant absorption due to non-pulsatile
arterial, venous and capillary blood

Absorption due to bone,
tissue, and other pigments

Figure 64. Components of the pulse oximeter waveform.

Oxygen content and oxygen tension measurement

Definitions

- **Oxygen content**: oxygen bound by haemoglobin + oxygen dissolved in solution. Measured as volume at STP or molecular mass (the relationship between volume at STP and mass is constant, see Avogadro's law).
- The **amount** of oxygen bound by haemoglobin depends on haemoglobin concentration, its oxygen-carrying capacity and oxygen saturation. The first and last factors are variable. Oxygen carrying capacity is fairly constant.
- **Oxygen tension**: partial pressure of oxygen in solution (pO_2). Measured in units of pressure (mmHg or kPa).
- **Oxygen concentration**: strictly speaking applies only to concentration in a gaseous mixture (e.g. air has 21% oxygen). Sometimes applied to oxygen content.
- **Oxygen saturation**: oxygen content/oxygen carrying capacity. See pulse oximetry and oxygen dissociation curve.

Oxygen content measurement

Physical method: van Slyke (Figure 65)

This is a **manometric** method. Instead of volume the apparatus **measures pressure** at constant volume and temperature. Change in pressure then accurately reflects change in the mass of gas (Avogadro's and Boyle's laws apply).

Oxygen has to be released from the blood sample by haemolysing the red cells with saponin and treating haemoglobin with ferricyanide to convert it to methaemoglobin – this releases all oxygen bound to haemoglobin. At the same time, CO_2 is released by the application of lactic acid. The released gases are extracted into vacuum and compressed to a standard volume. Vacuum extraction and subsequent compression is done by the means of lowering and raising the mercury levelling bulb. The gases are absorbed in turn (oxygen with sodium hydrosulphite, CO_2 with sodium hydroxide) and the resulting change in pressure measured. The burette is surrounded by a water jacket for temperature maintenance; temperature is measured and adjusted for standard temperature.

The apparatus is glass and is therefore breakable; the method is slow and cumbersome but very accurate. It is suitable for calibration of other analysers.

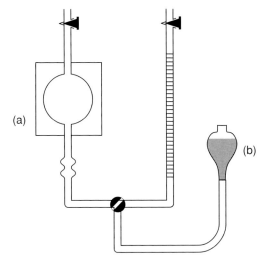

(a)

(b)

Figure 65. Van Slyke apparatus (a) water jacket; (b) mercury levelling bulb. Reproduced with permission from Butterworth-Heinemann.

Electrochemical method: fuel cell (Figure 66a)

This method uses the oxygen reaction with water and an electric current (the electron is denoted as e^-).

$$O_2 + 4e^- + 2H_2O \rightarrow 4(OH)^-.$$

The amount of **current** consumed in the above reaction is directly proportional to the rate of reduction of oxygen at the cathode, and since the only source of oxygen in the fuel cell was the blood sample introduced, the ampermeter readout, after electronic integration, will give oxygen content. Temperature compensation needs to be applied by means of a thermistor.

The fuel cell is a **battery** and has, therefore, a limited life. External voltage need not be applied as the battery produces its own. The amount of oxygen used in the reaction depends on oxygen uptake at the cathode and thus on its **partial pressure**. To obtain the oxygen bound in haemoglobin in solution, oxygen has to be released from haemoglobin. This is done in an apparatus, called Lex-O_2-Con, by haemolyzing the blood sample with distilled water in a scrubber and passing oxygen-free carrier gas through it. The carrier gas is nitrogen with 1% CO. The CO reacts with haemoglobin in a similar manner as ferricyanide in the van Slyke apparatus, i.e. it releases all the oxygen. Oxygen partial pressure in the carrier gas then directly corresponds to the concentration in solution as the gaseous and liquid phase are in equilibrium.

Polarographic method: Clark electrode (Figure 66b)

This method uses the same electrochemical reaction as described above. However, no battery is incorporated and therefore an **external voltage** of 0.6V must be applied. Note that electrodes are different – a platinum cathode and silver/silver chloride anode. Current flow is then measured which, as in the case above, depends on oxygen tension at the platinum cathode.

The cathode is protected from deposits by a thin plastic membrane; this separates it from the blood sample, and blood equilibrates with a small amount of electrolyte surrounding the cathode. Temperature is again controlled at $37\,^\circ C$.

This method is commonly used in **blood gas analysers**. The oxygen electrode must be kept clean and the plastic membrane regularly checked for deposits or puncture and then replaced.

Paramagnetic method (Figure 67)

This technique uses oxygen paramagnetic properties (oxygen is **attracted** into a magnetic field). This is because the electrons in the outer shell of an oxygen molecule are unpaired. Most other gases, e.g. nitrogen, are diamagnetic (repelled from a magnetic field).

The gas analyser contains a gastight chamber with a glass dumb-bell filled with nitrogen, which is suspended on a filament. A non-uniform magnetic field is applied across the chamber. When oxygen is introduced into the chamber, it displaces the glass dumb-bell filled with nitrogen (as oxygen is attracted into the magnetic field, while nitrogen is repelled). This displacement can be measured because the dumb-bell rotates on the filament. A mirror attached

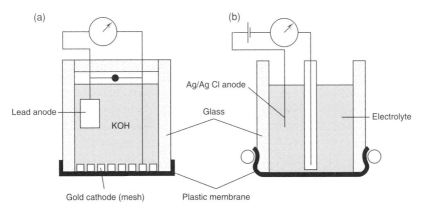

Figure 66. Oxygen measurement: (a) fuel cell (b) Clarke electrode. Reproduced with permission from Butterworth-Heinemann.

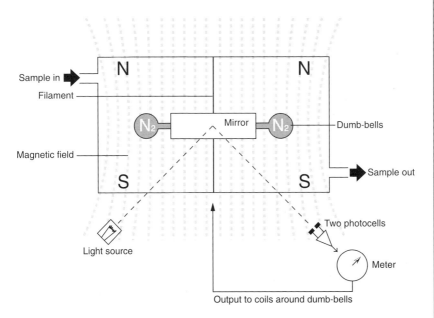

Figure 67. Paramagnetic oxygen analyser.

to the dumb-bell reflects a light beam and in older versions indicated the position on a calibrated scale. In the newer **null-deflection** system two photocells receive the light beam – their output is compared and used to generate a current around the dumb-bell which produces an opposing magnetic field and thus keeps the dumb-bell in its resting position. This apparatus is very accurate and fast; it is used in most modern on-line anaesthetic gas analysers for breath-by-breath analysis.

Mass spectrometry (Figure 68)

This method can be used for measurement of any gas. It separates gases according to their **molecular weight**.

A gas sample introduced is ionized and the ions are then separated, based on their respective **charge-to-mass** (Q/m) ratio. Only a small amount is analysed, which diffuses into the system via a molecular leak. Ionization is achieved by bombarding the sample with electrons. Separating can be done by means of eliminating all ions except those with a specific Q/m ratio. This happens in the **quadrupole** system: the electrical potential across the four rods is varied so that the ions oscillate as they travel. As the oscillations increase, the ions hit the rods and lose their charge; only the measured gas is allowed to travel through. In a **sector** system, the separating is done by means of a magnetic field applied across the flow of ions; these are then deflected according to their Q/m ratio and the deflected beams collected in specific positions in collector 'cups'.

This instrument allows rapid simultaneous breath-by-breath analysis of respiratory gases and vapours. It is used in the latest gas analysers. Its cost is prohibitive for day-to-day use but it is useful for research purposes. Size is no longer a problem; a portable system has been developed.

In summary, paramagnetic and mass spectrometric methods are suitable for analysis of respiratory gas mixtures; van Slyke, fuel cell and polarographic methods are suitable for blood gas analysis.

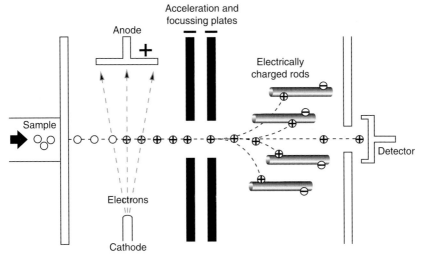

Figure 68. Quadruple mass spectrometer.

Capnography

Capnography is the measurement of carbon dioxide in a gas mixture. It uses the method of **infrared absorption spectrophotometry**. All gases with dissmilar atoms in the molecule, such as carbon dioxide and nitrous oxide, absorb infrared light. Peak absorbance by carbon dioxide is at 4.26 μm, fairly close to, but distinguishable from, the two nitrous oxide peaks at a slightly higher wavelength. Modern capnographs therefore utilize narrow bandwidth infrared light of 4.26 μm wavelength. Figure 69 shows as schematic representation of a capnograph. After passing through the monochromatic filter and the sampling chamber, residual light is detected by an infrared light detector and processed electronically. The windows of the sampling chamber have to be made from halogen crystals or other materials that do not absorb infrared light. To avoid drift, most instruments incorporate a reference chamber and a chopper close to the source of light to provide a discontinuous source of light (not included in the diagram).

There are two types of infrared CO_2 monitors: sidestream and mainstream capnographs; they differ in the gas sampling technique. Sidestream capnographs sample from the breathing system via a sampling line. The apparatus is lightweight and is suitable after adaptation for unintubated subjects. Mainstream capnographs have a measuring head placed in close proximity to the endotracheal tube, and the measuring chamber is heated to prevent condensation. These are heavy and cumbersome, are sensitive to external contamination with dirt and have the potential to cause burns and to break. However, they have a faster response time, less scope for error and are unaffected by expiratory flow rate.

A problem common to both types is response time – the signal is a saturation exponential function of time with a time constant about 0.1 s. Therefore a 90% response time is achieved in about 0.2 s (two time constants). Most capnographs can then cope with respiratory rates up to 60 min^{-1} but if further delay is introduced by a long sampling line, inaccuracies can occur at rates of 40 min^{-1}.

Waveform analysis (5 mm s^{-1})

In Figure 70, a single-breath gas washout curve is depicted. Phase I between points A and B represents dead space gas, in which there is no CO_2, unless it is being added (dead space gas is the fresh gas). After a rapid rise, points B–C or phase II, the end-tidal CO_2 curve reaches the alveolar plateau – points C–D (phase III), which is often sloping slightly upwards because of uneven emptying of different alveolar regions with varying time constants, and because the lung volume is getting progressively smaller, whereas CO_2 excretion continues. A further increase may occur at the end between points D and E (phase IV), if expiration proceeds below closing capacity.

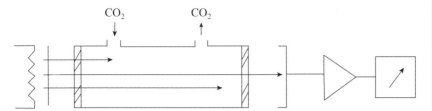

Figure 69. Principal components of a capnograph.
From left to right: infrared light source, filter, sampling chamber, light detector, processor, output.

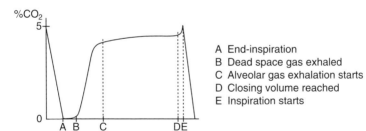

A End-inspiration
B Dead space gas exhaled
C Alveolar gas exhalation starts
D Closing volume reached
E Inspiration starts

Figure 70. Single breath analysis.

Abnormalities of single breath waveform (see Figure 71)

(a) Steep phase III as shown in Figure 71a. Alveolar emptying is more uneven. This happens in asthma or chronic obstructive airways disease, and is due to different time constants in different lung regions with various degrees of altered compliance and airways resistance.

(b) Cardiogenic oscillations (Figure 71b). This may happen in paediatric circuits, during low anaesthesia, and at low respiratory rates. In these cases, gas sampling rate exceeds expiratory flow. The 'ripples' are caused by cardiac activity and pulmonary blood flow. The oscillations can be eliminated by application of positive end-expiratory pressure or moving sampling port most distally.

(c) Dip in alveolar plateau (usually only seen in ventilated patients). The dip means the patient makes a small inspiratory effort during the course of expiration. Action by the anaesthetist will depend on the stage of operation and postoperative plan.

(d) Rebreathing (Figure 71d). The capnographic waveform does not return to zero on inspiration and gradually shift upwards, with a same or higher amplitude. Rebreathing is eliminated by removing dead space.

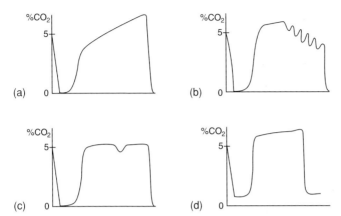

Figure 71. Abnormalities of single breath curve, (a) chronic obstructive airways disease, (b) cardiogenic oscillations, (c) dip in plateau, (d) rebreathing.

Trend analysis (display at 25 mm min^{-1})

Hypercapnia (end-tidal only)

As shown in Figure 72 can be caused by:

(a) Increased CO_2 production (pyrexia) or a sudden CO_2 load (release of tourniquets or aortic clamp, i.v. bicarbonate, insufflation of CO_2). Reduced CO_2 elimination – depression of respiratory centre, or reduction of ventilation due to neuromuscular problems or iatrogenic (IPPV).

(b) Baseline drift upward from zero indicates rebreathing or a calibration error: compare the two graphs of hypercapnia.

Hypocapnia (Figure 73)

(a) Increased CO_2 elimination – hyperventilation (common cause): slow exponential fall.

(b) Decreased CO_2 production – hypothermia: slow exponential fall. Major disturbance to pulmonary or systemic circulation (shock, air embolism, cardiac malfunction): fast exponential fall in end-tidal CO_2.

(c) Endotracheal tube kinking or disconnection: abrupt fall.

In the last two situations, end-tidal CO_2 does not accurately reflect arterial p_{CO_2}. The p_aCO_2–ETCO$_2$ gradient will then be increased over the usual 2–3 mmHg (5 mmHg in anaesthetized subjects).

Uses of capnography

- Confirmation of endotracheal intubation (oesophageal intubation false-positive only in first few breaths).
- During IPPV to determine the correct level of minute ventilation.
- During anaesthesia with spontaneous breathing to monitor respiratory activity, determine fresh gas flow and anaesthetic agent requirement (in particular during low flow).
- Detection of disconnection.
- Trend analysis as above.
- Differential diagnosis of hypotension (induced hypotension versus cardiovascular collapse).

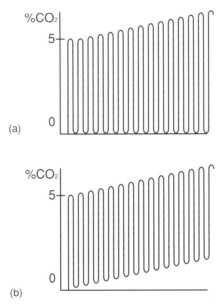

Figure 72. (a) Hypercapnia:(a) carbon dioxide overproduction or absorption, (b) rebreathing.

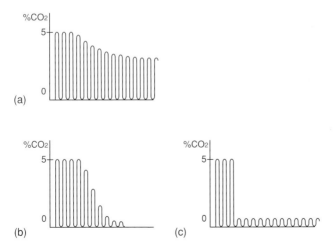

Figure 73. Hypocapnia (a) overventilation, (b) collapse, (c) disconnection.

[H$^+$], pH and its measurement

Basics of acid–base balance

Maximum strength of acid $= 1$ g/l [H$^+$] ($= 10^0$ g/l). Maximum strength of alkali $= 10^{-14}$ g/l [H$^+$]. Water is halfway between 10^0 and $10^{-14} = 10^{-7}$ g/l $= 100$ nmol/l (1 nmol $= 10^{-9}$ mol).

To make these small numbers easier to handle, and to accommodate the large range, Sorensen proposed a logarithmic scale, so that

$$pH = -\log_{10}[H^+].$$

For the definition of a logarithm, see the chapter on exponentials. The logarithmic scale has equal distances between the powers of 10, or 'e' in the case of natural logarithms, rather than between the units. It converts an exponential curve into a straight line, as can be seen in Figure 74. For the effect of a logarithmic scale on the population distribution of hydrogen ion concentration and pH, see the chapter on statistics.

The physiological concentration of H$^+$ is near water but slightly on the alkaline side: 40 nmol/l. Thus physiological pH $= -\log_{10} 40 \times 10^{-9}$:

$$= -\log_{10} 4 \times 10^{-8} = -(0.6 - 8) = -(-7.4) =$$
$$= 7.4.$$

The normal pH range is 7.36–7.44, i.e. very narrow. pH < 7 is already a severe acidosis.

When converting [H$^+$] to pH, we have to appreciate the properties of the logarithmic scale. While small changes into the alkaline direction of hydrogen ion concentration result in significant changes in pH, the reverse happens on the acid side: between pH 8 and 7, the H ion concentration changes 10-fold, 10–100 nmol/l; between pH 7 and 6, the H ion concentration changes 10-fold again, 100–1000 nmol/l, while the pH only lost another unit. Figure 73 shows this relationship between the pH values of 6 and 8. Bold linear scale on the x-axis relates to the bold exponential curve. The scale of the logarithmic x-axis is arbitrarily chosen to fit of [H$^+$] 40 and 100.

In practice, pH users know that pH about 6 is an extremely severe metabolic acidosis, and are not fooled by the seemingly small change in pH. Furthermore, on the alkaline side the physiological consequences of a smaller deviation are equally devastating, i.e. severe metabolic alkalosis, or perhaps more, since the body is not well equipped to deal with an alkali load (or [H$^+$] deficit); the change on the alkaline side in hydrogen ion concentration from 40 to 10 nmol appears rather small and belies the seriousness of the condition.

A practical way for an approximate conversion of [H$^+$] into pH follows from the properties of the exponential curve: for each 0.3 change in pH between 7 and 8, halve the hydrogen ion concentration (from 100 at 7 to 12.5 at 7.9); for each 0.3 unit change in pH between 7 and 6, double the hydrogen ion concentration (from 100 at 7 to 800 at 6.1). The numbers are not exact because the factor of 0.3 is not exact.

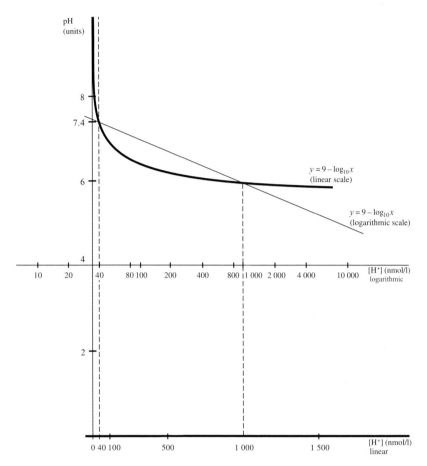

Figure 74. [H$^+$]–pH relationship on a linear and logarithmic scale.

It is possible to argue that because physiological processes of elimination tend to happen exponentially, perhaps using pH makes more sense than the H ion concentration. It would have been even more logical to use natural logarithms. These are not, however, easy to handle mathematically. Notice that the pH electrode reacts in direct proportion to pH, not $[H^+]$.

pH meter (Figure 75)

The instrument is a potentiometer, i.e. measures change in electrical **potential** across two electrodes. It acts as a **battery**, i.e. no electromagnetic force (voltage) need be applied. The Hg/HgCl electrode is a reference electrode that maintains a constant electromagnetic potential. The Ag/AgCl electrode is the pH electrode and incorporates pH-sensitive glass: the potential across the glass changes in direct proportion to unit pH (not $[H^+]$ – another example of a natural exponential process), i.e. 60 mV per unit pH. When the sample chamber is empty the battery is 'disconnected'. When a blood sample is introduced the circuit is completed and the potential can be measured across the two electrodes.

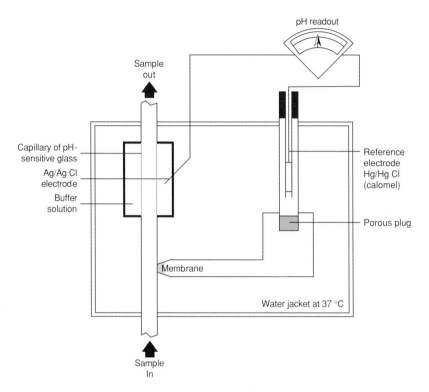

pH readout

Sample
out

Capillary of pH-
sensitive glass

Ag/Ag Cl
electrode

Buffer
solution

Reference
electrode
Hg/Hg Cl
(calomel)

Porous plug

Membrane

Water jacket at 37 °C

Sample
In

Figure 75. The pH electrode. Reproduced with permission from Butterworth-Heinemann.

2 | Principles of measurement of flow in gases and liquids

Flow measurement is based on the physical principles underlying the definition of flow.

$$Q = A.v$$

In words, **flow** is measured as a **function of velocity** (for an illustration, see the chapter on laminar flow). This principle is used, for instance, in the **electromagnetic flowmeter**: electric potential develops across a magnetic field through which blood is moving; the magnitude of this potential is directly proportional to the average velocity of blood flow. **Ultrasonic flowmeters** use the change in frequency of an audio signal when it is reflected from moving red blood cells. This again depends on blood velocity. If the diameter of the vessels is measured at the same time, blood flow is computed and displayed simultaneously.

Two methods of gas flow measurement are based on this formula:

$$Q = \Delta p / R$$

- **Variable orifice** (and thus resistance), **constant pressure**. **Flow** is then inversely **related to resistance** or directly related to the size of the orifice. Laminar flow increases 16 times if the radius of the orifice doubles (see the chapter on flow). Conversely, flow is reduced 16 times when the radius is halved and two times if the radius is only 15% less. In Figure 76, water (rather than gas) flow from a mains pipe with a tap is plotted against the resistance offered by the tap. It is shown that closing the tap only slightly from the maximum at point A, to reduce its diameter by 15% at point B, halves the flow. The Rotameter and the Wright peak flow meter are examples of variable orifice flowmeters. Constant pressure in the former is provided by the pressure of the bobbin; the pressure is the ratio of the product of the mass and gravity over the cross sectional area of the bobbin ($p = F/A = m\, a/A$). The Rotameter is tapered, and thus the magnitude of the orifice around the bobbin corresponds to the magnitude of gas flow. In Wright's peak flow meter the opposing pressure is the tension from a coiled spring acting on the rotating vane area.
- **Constant orifice** (and resistance), **variable pressure**. The **flow** in this case is **directly proportional to the pressure** drop ($Q = R^{-1}\Delta p$, where $R = $ constant), i.e. a linear relationship (Figure 77). The pneumotachograph is based on this method: a pressure drop across a gauze screen or a light, plastic valve of known resistance is measured and transduced. In Figure 75, the relationship between pressure and flow is illustrated as flow from a vessel with a fixed outlet resistance. The magnitude of flow at any given moment is directly proportional to the hydrostatic pressure in the vessel. Pressure is higher at point B on the plot, and flow is correspondingly higher. (The sequence of events in practice would be from point B to point A.)

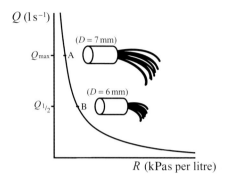

Figure 76. Reciprocal relationship between flow and resistance for constant pressure.

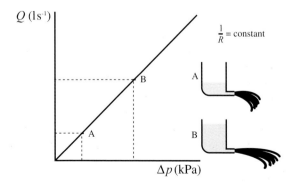

Figure 77. Linear relationship between driving pressure and flow.

$Q = dV/dt$

Flow as the rate of change of volume with time. 'd' means change or derivative. Cardiac output by the thermal dilution method uses this formula (see the next chapter).

It may be helpful to define the derivative and the reverse process, integration at this point. The **derivative** is the **slope of the tangent to the curve representing a given function**. It is described as the rate of change of the function.

Figure 78 illustrates **constant flow** as a derivative. Volume of mains water that passed through the area of interest (the measurement point) is plotted against time. The flow of water through a pipe under mains pressure is constant, and the rate of rise of volume collected with time is constant: over 1 s, we collect, say, 100 ml, over 1 min, 6000 ml. When volume against time is plotted, the **slope** of this linear relationship is also the slope of the derivative, the flow. Its numerical value is given by the fraction V_t/t; this is constant at any point on the line: the flow is constant.

Exponentially falling flow, such as when emptying a bath, is the subject of the chapter on exponentials.

If we chart flow and wish to know what the volume collected was over a specified time, **integration** is applied. Derivation of volume with time yielded flow; integration of flow, the reverse operation, yields volume. Calculation of volume from flow is easily done by multiplication of the flow by the specified time. Mathematically and graphically this is called integration: a small volume passed in a unit of time can be depicted as the area of a small rectangle with sides equal to the two variables (unit of time and increment of volume over time i.e. flow). In Figure 79 the rectangles under the line of flow are the individual increments. As the flow is constant, it is obvious that the sum of these incremental rectangles is equal to the total area under the line. If the flow were variable e.g. decreasing such as in Figure 80, and the incremental rectangles infinitely narrow, so that the irregularity of the curve at the top of the rectangle is minimised, their sum would again be equal to the **area under the curve** (AUC). To sum up **integration with respect to time is summation of increments over time in order to obtain total**.

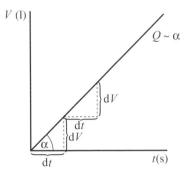

Figure 78. Flow as a derivative of volume with respect to time.

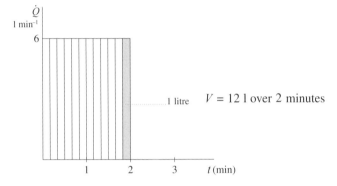

$V = 12\,\mathrm{l}$ over 2 minutes

Figure 79. Area under the line of flow = volume passed. Constant flow.

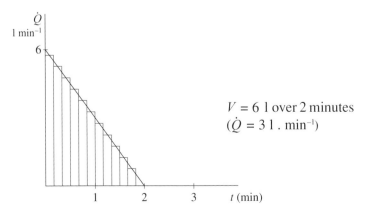

$V = 6\,\mathrm{l}$ over 2 minutes
$(\dot{Q} = 3\,\mathrm{l}.\ \mathrm{min}^{-1})$

Figure 80. Decreasing flow.

Principles of measurement of flow in gases and liquids

Cardiac output measurement by thermal dilution technique

Bedside cardiac output measurement (Figure 81) using the thermal dilution technique is based on the formula $Q = dV/dt$.

It is the measurement of blood volume that passed the measuring point during one circulation time.

Since collection of aortic blood flow over any period is not a bedside option, the blood volume that passed over the measurement period is measured indirectly, as a change in blood temperature, or 'concentration of cold'. A known quantity of cold saline is injected into the bloodstream and is thus mixed with circulating blood, reducing its temperature. The volume of the saline (10 ml) is negligible compared with the diluting volume and does not require correction in the calculation. The 'quantity of cold', or negative heat, is also small but it is sufficiently large to produce a measurable temperature drop, which of course changes with time as the mixing is done in the bloodstream. Blood temperature is recorded intravascularly with a thermistor at the tip of the pulmonary artery flotation catheter, and the signal is processed by computer.

Remember there is a **reciprocal relationship between volume and concentration**. In other words, what we measure (concentration of cold) is inversely related to the result (blood flow). The diluting blood volume calculated as the ratio of 'mass' of cold and concentration of cold ($V = $ m/c) is then used in the formula above for the calculation of cardiac output:

$$V = m/c$$

To know the final hypothetical 'concentration of cold', the cardiac computer applies integration (see the previous chapter): integration of the instantaneous change in concentration (dc/dt) yields total final concentration over specified time, t. The integral, as shown in the previous chapter, is the area under the curve (AUC) of the instantaneous recording in the concentration. The **reciprocal relationship between cardiac output and AUC** still applies, as we merely substitute AUC for 'concentration of cold' in the volume formula:

$$V(\text{diluting volume}) = m/c = \text{amount of cold/AUC}$$

Cardiac output is then calculated by substituting the result, diluting volume, V, which is the volume of one circulation, into the flow formula.

In Figure 81, the instantaneous change in blood temperature is shown with its mirror image, the 'concentration of cold'. The lower curve is the familiar shape produced on the cardiac computer screen. Remember that the curve is not the pulmonary artery flow but the concentration of cold saline, the 'blip' on it is not the dicrotic notch but the change in temperature with recirculation, and the area under it is not cardiac output but a hypothetical final concentration of cold saline. Because of recirculation the first large curve must be extrapolated to zero and the area under this curve only is calculated.

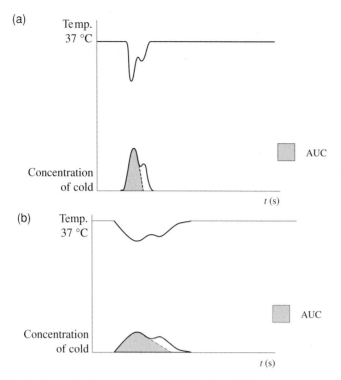

Figure 81. Cardiac output measurement (a) high output, (b) low output.

The AUC is identical for the temperature and 'concentration' curves for a particular cardiac output. Compare the 'high output' graph with the 'low output' one: the peak of the low output curve is smaller but the total AUC is larger. This makes sense if we keep in mind that a fast flow will produce a swiftly rising and falling concentration curve, with a greater instantaneous change in temperature but a small AUC, while slow flow will do the opposite.

2 Measurement of the mechanical properties of the chest

Static compliance ($C = \Delta V / \Delta p$)

The change in volume is measured as the patient takes a breath from a **spirometer**.

A change in pressure is given as the difference between pleural and alveolar pressure. Direct pleural pressure measurement would produce a pneumothorax; **oesophageal pressure** is a good approximation. With the glottis open and after equilibration, the **mouth pressure** is (for measurement purposes) equal to alveolar pressure. The measurement is taken at different lung volumes, and compliance is calculated from the slope of the pressure/volume plot. See the chapter on respiratory mechanics for the plot.

Airways resistance ($R = \Delta p / Q = p_{alv} - p_{mouth}\ Q$)

The pressure gradient is the difference between alveolar and mouth pressures during flow.

Mouth pressure can be measured directly by a **pressure transducer**; alveolar pressure has to be derived, for instance, as a reciprocal value to a change in pressure inside an airtight box (**body plethysmograph**) during tidal breathing. In Figure 82, the pressure waveform of alveolar pressure and pressure inside the box are plotted against each other to show the relationship.

Flow is measured directly by a pneumotachograph, and resistance calculated.

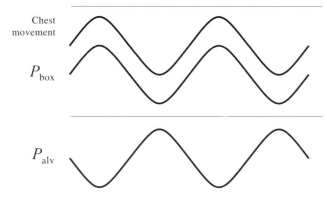

Chest
movement

P_{box}

P_{alv}

Figure 82. Pressure changes in constant volume plethysmograph.

Lung volumes and their measurement

Figure 83 shows the lung volumes. The 'capacities' are sums of individual volumes.

Tidal volume and the volumes above can be measured directly by a Benedict–Roth spirometer, not described here. The volumes below resting expiratory level are best measured indirectly.

Functional residual capacity (FRC)

The FRC is of more interest than residual volume, particularly the relationship of FRC to the closing volume. The indirect measurements utilize the principle of dilution of a known mass of a gas in the unknown volume.

Closed circuit helium

The closed circuit helium wash-in method employs this gas because it is relatively insoluble in blood: gas uptake is assumed to be zero. The patient rebreathes from a closed circuit with a known concentration of helium. CO_2 is absorbed and sufficient oxygen supplied for adequate oxygenation. After equilibration the mass, m, of helium in the volume composed of FRC and the volume of the apparatus, V, must be the same as the mass of helium which was originally in the apparatus only

$$m_1 = m_2$$
$$m = V c$$
$$V[He_1] = (FRC + V).[He_2].$$
$$\text{Therefore FRC} = V[He_1 - He_2]/He_2.$$

This is illustrated in Figure 84: a known volume of a known concentration of helium is mixed with the unknown volume (FRC). After mixing, the helium concentration in the total volume is lower (as there was no helium in FRC). Helium concentration is measured by a **katharometer** (a measurement apparatus based on the change of thermal conductivity).

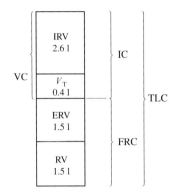

IRV – inspiratory reserve volume
VT – tidal volume
ERV – expiratory reserve volume
RV – residual volume
FRC – functional residual capacity
IC   – inpiratory capacity
VC – vital capacity
TLC – total lung capacity

Figure 83. Lung volumes.

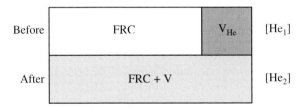

Figure 84. Measurement of functional residual capacity (FRC) by helium wash-in method.

Open circuit nitrogen washout

Open circuit nitrogen washout similarly employs nitrogen dilution in the lungs after a period of oxygen breathing. The exhaled volume has to be collected and measured. The mass of nitrogen found in the exhaled collected gas (calculated as the product of final expired concentration of nitrogen, f_E, and the sum of exhaled volume, V_E, plus the volume of the apparatus, V_{App}) must be the same as the mass of gas which left the lung (given by the product of FRC and the difference between alveolar concentration of nitrogen before and after the period of oxygen breathing, $f_{A1} - f_{A2}$):

$$(V_E + V_{App}).f_E = FRC.(f_{A1} - f_{A2}).$$
$$\text{Therefore } FRC = (V_E + V_{App}).f_E/f_{A1} - f_{A2}.$$

Figure 82 illustrates this situation. What is in effect done is mixing a known concentration of nitrogen (80%) from an unknown volume (FRC) into a larger volume (expired volume plus the volume of the apparatus), and the resulting concentration is measured. Because not all nitrogen is washed out, alveolar concentration of nitrogen at the end of oxygen breathing has to be subtracted from the alveolar concentration at the beginning. Alveolar concentration is assumed to equal end-tidal concentration of nitrogen. During oxygen breathing, nitrogen is also being washed out from blood and the tissues; this proceeds more slowly and is not taken into account.

The above methods can also be used to determine the **distribution of inspired air**. Poorly aerated lung zones have long time constants to achieve equilibrium when gas composition is changed. With helium wash-in, the number of breaths needed to achieve equilibrium is the measure of the time elapsed (15–30 breaths, or <3 min). Control measurement is needed to compensate for the characteristics of the apparatus. Nitrogen washout takes longer; in normal lungs alveolar concentration of nitrogen after 7 min is < 2.5%. Values greater than this indicate non-uniform distribution of inspired gas.

Dead space volume, closing volume (single breath analysis of expired nitrogen)

During and after a single breath of oxygen, the change in volume is plotted against time, and simultaneously nitrogen concentration in expired air is monitored.

In Figure 83, the volume plot against time is shown in the upper half, and expired nitrogen concentration in the lower half. During inspiration of oxygen, nitrogen concentration will be zero; it stays at zero while dead space gas is breathed out. When alveolar gas reaches the measuring point, nitrogen concentration abruptly rises and stays at a plateau for most of the expiration. Towards the end of expiration, when closing volume is reached, it rises again, as more concentrated nitrogen is breathed out from a smaller lung volume. Dead space volume and closing volume can simply be read from the plot between the points indicated.

In a patient with emphysema and a high physiological dead space, the alveolar plateau of nitrogen is never reached – nitrogen concentration continues to increase from the beginning of expiration until the end.

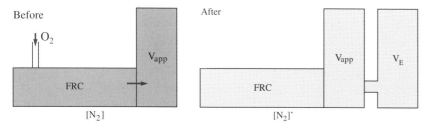

Figure 85. Measurement of functional residual capacity (FRC) by nitrogen washout.

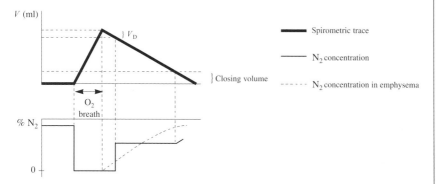

Figure 86. Single breath nitrogen washout. Reproduced with permission from Butterworth-Heinemann.

Part 3a

Physiology: the cardiovascular system

The cardiac cycle and the intravascular pressure waveforms

With the exception of systemic arterial pressure, intravascular pressure waveforms can be observed during pulmonary artery catheterization.

The balloon-tipped catheter is introduced into a central vein and with appropriate scale adjustment the **central venous pressure trace**, similar to the one opposite, can be seen. The A wave corresponds to atrial contraction, and is followed by the C wave: tricuspid valve closure simultaneous with ventricular contraction. X descent follows, as the right atrium and central vein are now empty and ventricular pressure is now indirectly transmitted across the valve. The right atrium starts filling until the tricuspid valve opens again. The V wave corresponds to the valve opening, following which central venous pressure drops momentarily (the Y descent) as the right atrium empties passively into the right ventricle until the next atrial systole.

The scale is usually adjusted to monitor right ventricular pressures, and the central venous pressure trace is then an undulating waveform around the usual 6–8 mmHg. A straight line indicates a technical problem such as wrong connection or a kinked line.

At 15 cm the balloon is inflated and the catheter advanced downstream. After 20 cm the catheter should enter the right atrium. **Right atrial pressure** is related to central venous pressure, their difference being the hydrostatic pressure difference; in the supine patient this difference is very small.

Right ventricular pressure trace is instantly recognized when the systolic pressure reaches 20–25 mmHg, while the diastolic pressure should be close to zero.

At about 30 cm, the catheter tip should pass the pulmonary valve and the **pulmonary artery pressure** trace should be seen. Its shape and amplitude are similar to the ventricular pressure trace; however, the effect of the pulmonary valve closure can be seen as the pressure trace does not return to zero, and the diastolic pressure is about 8–12 mmHg.

Figure 87 shows a semi-diagrammatic representation of several related parameters on the right side of the heart.

For better illustration, heart sounds are added to relate the pressure recordings to the mechanical events (valve closures), and an ECG waveform to relate these events to the electrical cycle.

Note how the pulmonary artery systolic pressure is identical with the right ventricular systolic pressure; the difference between these pressures is in the diastolic pressure. Pulmonary artery occlusion pressure is not shown here, as this is a measurement relating to the left side of the heart.

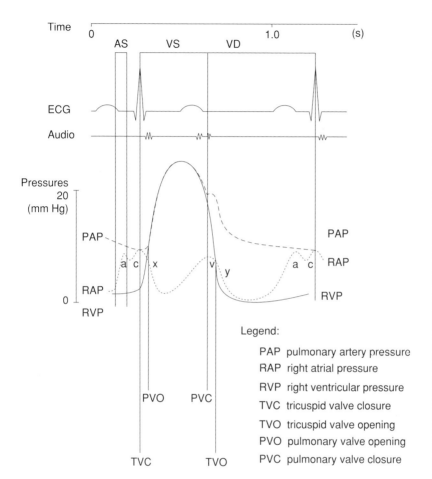

Figure 87. Intravascular pressure waveforms on the right side of the heart during pulmonary artery catheterisation. Adapted from: C. G. Caro, T. J. Pedioy, R. C. Schroter & W. A. Seed, *The Mechanics of Circulation*, OUP, 1978.

After a further 5–10 cm, the balloon occludes the pulmonary artery and a continuous column of blood should exist between the catheter tip and the left atrium. A pressure trace now recorded is the **pulmonary artery occlusion pressure** ('wedge pressure'). This corresponds to left atrial pressure and left ventricular filling pressure, provided the following conditions are fulfilled

- The pulmonary intravascular pressure exceeds extravascular pressure, to obtain a continuous column of blood. This condition is not fulfilled if the intravascular pressure is low, e.g. when the catheter is lodged in West zone 1, or if the extravascular pressure is abnormally high, as with the application of positive end-expiratory pressure.
- The pressure in the left atrium reflects the left ventricular end-diastolic pressure (LVEDP). In mitral valve disease left atrial pressure can be much higher than LVEDP. Conversely, in heart failure when sinus rhythm is preserved, LVEDP may be higher than the mean left atrial pressure: left atrial pressure increases to the high ventricular level only during the atrial systole.

Wedging of the pulmonary artery flotation catheter can be seen on the screen as a sudden decrease in the amplitude of the pressure waveform to < 12 mmHg. (Left heart filling pressure is higher than on the right side.) On deflation of the balloon, a normal pulmonary artery trace should be seen again.

Arterial pressure waveform is shown in Figure 88 with airway pressure during intermittent positive pressure ventilation. Blood pressure trace shows changes in phase with respiration, called the **respiratory swing**. (For more details of the effects of intermittent positive pressure ventilation on blood pressure see next chapter.) As the intrathoracic pressure is only increased briefly during inspiration, overall effect is a decrease in arterial systolic and diastolic pressure which lags behind the increase in intrathroacic pressure. Respiratory swing is pronounced in hypovolaemia, and is a valuable tool in the estimation of fluid deficit. Notice also that the dicrotic notch is low and the arterial pressure trace is narrow in hypovolaemia. Many ITU monitors have different sweep speeds for arterial pressure and for respiration; association of blood pressure swing and airway pressure is then not observed on the monitor.

Arterial
blood pressure

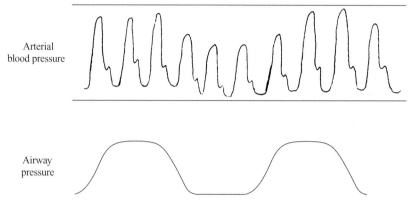

Airway
pressure

Figure 88. Arterial blood pressure and respiratory swing.

Cardiovascular effects of intermittent positive pressure ventilation

Intermittent positive pressure ventilation causes changes in intrathoracic pressure and blood volume, which are reflected in the cardiovascular parameters. Four phases can be recognized (see Figure 89):

- **Phase I**: blood is forced into the left atrium by the increased intrathoracic pressure – blood pressure rises and reflex bradycardia follows.
- **Phase IIa**: blood pressure falls because of decreased venous return – the result of the raised intrathoracic pressure.
- **Phase IIb**: blood pressure is restored to normal by reflex tachycardia.
- **Phase III**: venous return is decreased on lowering the intrathoracic pressure as there is now increased venous capacity in the lungs. Blood pressure falls initially but normalizes soon as reflex tachycardia persists.
- **Phase IV**: persisting tachycardia results in an overshoot of blood pressure; heart rate then drops back to normal (baroreceptor reflex) and blood pressure then also normalizes.

The magnitude of the effect on blood pressure as a result of effects on right and left ventricular filling depends on **blood volume** and the **integrity of the sympathetic nervous system** control, i.e. effects will be exaggerated in the presence of hypovolaemia, sympathetic blockade (this includes general anaesthesia) or autonomic dysfunction (e.g. diabetic neuropathy), or a combination of factors (ill patients, e.g. sepsis), as compensation is lost ('blocked Valsalva'). The ventilator settings also play a role – fast ventilation rates with a long inspiratory phase will allow little time for compensation; high ventilation pressures will cause greater effects.

In patients with pulmonary hypertension (e.g. severe ARDS), increased airway pressure during intermittent positive pressure ventilation results in increased pulmonary vascular resistance. Interventricular septum may shift to the left and compromise the left ventricular filling, and eventually decrease the stroke volume. Because the lung is leaky in ARDS, inspiration pressure has to be controlled rather than fluids administered to improve left ventricular filling.

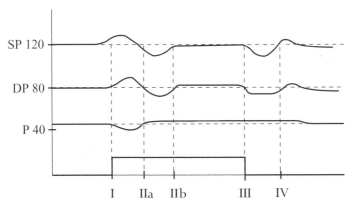

Figure 89. Arterial blood pressure and pulse during the Valsalva manoeuvre. SP, DP – systolic and diastolic pressures. P – pulse.

Control of cardiac output, regulation of cardiac function

Cardiac output is the product of **stroke volume and heart rate**. Both are under the control of the **sympathetic nervous system**. Stroke volume is also affected by changes in **preload, contractility** and **afterload**, and their inter-action. This chapter will deal with preload and afterload only. For the effect of contractility on cardiac performance, see chapter Cardiac cycle: pressure–volume relationships. **Venous return** (preload) depends on *blood volume, posture and venous tone*. Venous tone is under the control of the sympathetic nervous system. Sympathetic output changes in response to the peripheral metabolic need.

Figure 90 shows the **Frank–Starling relationship** between the left ven-tricular end-diastolic pressure (LVEDP) and stroke volume (SV). The Frank–Starling curve mechanism allows a ventricle to match its output (stroke vol-ume) to the volume of blood that enters it (the **preload**).

On the *x*-axis, end diastolic pressure is substituted for fibre length, and on the *y*-axis stroke volume is substituted for force of contraction (fibre length and force of contraction were the variables used in the original research on isolated muscle fibre). In practice, we use surrogate parameters that can be directly measured and make assumptions which are valid under normal phys-iological conditions, the assumption being that LVEDV (left ventricular end diastolic volume) $\sim$ LVEDP $=$ LAP (left atrial pressure) $=$ PAOP (pul-monary artery occlusion pressure). The relationship between LVEDP and SV is linear up to a certain unphysiological point. After that, the mechanism fails (in the original research this happened because of fibre disruption).

Point OP on the middle curve represents the operating point under 'nor-mal' conditions, with a filling pressure of about 8 mmg Hg and a stroke volume of 70 ml. The curves to the right and left show how the relationship changes under varying conditions of inotropy and **afterload**. The slope of the curve is increased with increasing inotropy or decrease in afterload. Conversely, the slope is less steep (the curve moves down) with increased afterload or a loss of inotropy.

In critically ill patients, we optimize the preload first in order to improve cardiac performance. Patients in circulatory failure due to volume loss will need generous levels of preload for optimum cardiac function. Patients in shock because of pump failure (e.g. myocardial infarction, chronic heart fail-ure) will need cautious filling to lower targets and a may need a reduction in afterload. Septic shock is a mixture of pump failure due to myocardial depression, and volume loss (absolute – due to pyrexia, or relative – due to vasodilatation); optimizing the preload is often a result of a trial and error process. Volume filling is done in small increments whilst at the same time manipulating the systemic vascular resistance to counter vasodilatation.

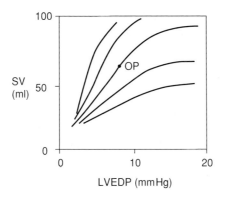

Figure 90. Frank–Starling curves. Changes in afterload and inotropy shift the Frank–Starling curve up or down.

Cardiac cycle: pressure–volume relationships

Left ventricular compliance and elastance

The heart fills during the diastole by venous return, augmented, if the heart is in sinus rhythm, by atrial contribution. The pressure–volume relationship in an object being filled is called **compliance** (dV/dp) – in this case the left ventricular compliance, left ventricular end-diastolic volume and left ventricular end-diastolic pressure.

In practice, ventricular pressures are more easily measured than ventricular volumes, and therefore the inverse of compliance, i.e. **elastance** or stiffness (dp/dV), is of interest. In Figure 91, the left ventricular pressure is chosen as the dependent variable, and the slope of the relationship between LVEDP and LVEDV corresponds to the stiffness of the left ventricle: the steeper the slope, the stiffer (less compliant, more thick walled or restricted) is the left ventricle. The relationship is linear up to a certain point of maximum stretch, beyond which the LVEDP rises steeply with any further increment of volume. Under physiological conditions, the heart operates on the linear part of the curve, and therefore it is possible to assume that LVEDP will correspond to LVEDV.

Note that the left ventricular end-diastolic volume corresponds to the initial fibre length of the Frank–Starling relationship. When measuring the pulmonary artery occlusion pressure (PAOP), we estimate the left ventricular filling from a pressure measurement inside a small pulmonary artery. The relationship between the PAOP and the LVEDV is complex (see more in chapter Control of cardiac output); ventricular compliance (or stiffness) is only one of the factors which can alter this relationship: a stiffer ventricle will achieve a smaller filling volume before the ventricle reaches the maximum capacity point, or conversely higher end-diastolic pressures are needed in order to achieve a comparable end-diastolic volume. This has to be borne in mind when interpreting the results of cardiac catheterization: the assumption that **left ventricular end-diastolic pressure** (estimated from the pulmonary artery occlusion pressure) **corresponds to left ventricular end-diastolic volume** only applies provided that left ventricular **compliance remains unaltered**.

Volatile anaesthetics decrease left ventricular compliance to various degrees, and this may be the basis for the extent to which they depress myocardial function.

The **left ventricle** maintains flow in the systemic circulation. It is a high-pressure system and, therefore, the left ventricle is thick walled.

The **right ventricle** and pulmonary circulation are a **low-pressure system**; the filling pressure is about 5 mmHg, and the systolic pressure about 20 mmHg. The ventricle is much more compliant than the left ventricle and thus can match left ventricular output at low pressures.

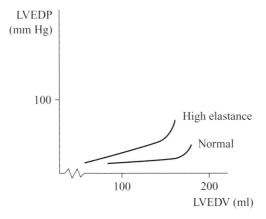

Figure 91. The relationship between left ventricular end-diastolic volume and end-diastolic pressure.

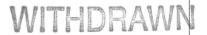

Pressure–volume loops

This is a dynamic representation of the relationship between left ventricular volume and left ventricular pressure during each phase of the cardiac cycle. The pressure volume loop can be used to describe **cardiac performance** and the effect of various changes in physiological parameters.

Starting from the ED (end-diastole) point in Figure 92(a), the left ventricle is filled to maximum and the ventricular systole starts. During the **isovolumetric phase** of the systole, **tension** develops in the muscle fibre which will relate to the force of contraction in the next phase. Ventricular volume during this phase remains unchanged.

During the **isotonic phase** of the systole, cardiac muscle contracts, i.e. **fibre shortening** occurs. The aortic valve opens and blood is ejected out of the ventricle. Ventricular pressure during this phase changes little until the ES (end-systolic) point, when it decrases abruptly as the ventricle relaxes during the isometric phase of the diastole.

The tangential line at the ES point describes the **end-systolic pressure–volume relationship** (ESPVR). Its slope corresponds to the inotropic state of the heart (see below).

The bottom line describes the pressure–volume relationship during the isotonic phase of diastole (ventricular filling). Its slope inversely relates to a particular state of ventricular **compliance**.

Figure 92b shows how the pressure–volume loop changes with an **increased state of inotropy**. Notice that the slope of the ESPVR is steeper, allowing the ventricle to contract more forcefully and therefore to increase the stroke volume (the difference between ES and ED point). The ES point therefore is lower on the x-axis (LV volume).

Figure 94c demonstrates the effect of **heart failure**. The slope of the ESPVR is lower, and the ventricle has to operate at a much higher filling volume in order to generate pressures comparable to 'normal' conditions. As emptying is inefficient, stroke volume is smaller and the ES point is much higher on the x-axis.

In acute heart failure due to myocardial depression such as occurs in septic shock, the heart has a relative lack of inotropic drive. The remedy in this case is to use inotropic infusion in order to improve the ESPVR and enable to ventricle to contract more efficiently. The loop will shift to the left ('normal').

By contrast, the efficiency of the heart in chronic heart failure or in states of high afterload can be improved by a decrease in afterload. This improves the slope of the Frank–Starling curve (see chapter Control of cardiac function), which improves the stroke volume for a given ventricular filling pressure. Thus the ES point and the whole loop moves left, and the ESPVR improves as a result.

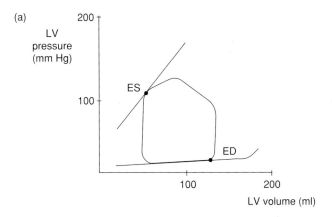

Figure 92(a). Left ventricular pressure–volume loop at steady-state.

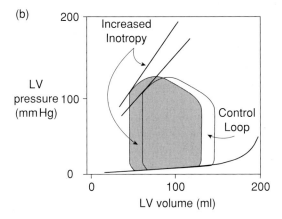

Figure 92(b). The effect of increased inotropy on left ventricular pressure–volume loop. Heart rate and aortic pressure held constant.

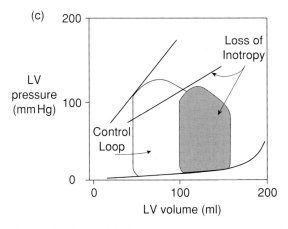

Figure 92(c). The effect of left ventricular failure (reduced inotropy) on left ventricular pressure–volume loop. Heart rate unchanged.

Blood pressure and blood volume relationship

Following blood loss, the body draws on its reserves to maintain blood flow and oxygen delivery to the tissues. Initially, water is retained by the kidney and extracellular fluid is drawn into the intravascular compartment. If blood loss continues, physiological compensatory mechanisms bring about changes in other physiological parameters to maintain blood flow to the tissues, and in a more severe haemorrhage to the vital organs only. Haemorrhage is classified into four degrees of severity:

- **Class I**: $\leq 15\%$ or ≤ 750 ml blood loss. Stroke volume may fall minimally at lower levels of loss, resulting in a minimal tachycardia to maintain cardiac output. This is the situation induced by venesection in a blood donor.
- **Class II**: 15–30% or 750–1500 ml blood loss. Tachycardia is noticeable while systolic blood pressure is still maintained; diastolic pressure, however, rises due to the higher level of circulating catecholamines. Mean blood pressure is maintained but flow to the organs without autoregulation of blood flow is reduced (e.g. muscle, skin). Because of the reduced skin blood flow, core-to-skin temperature difference starts to rise. Renal blood flow is minimally affected and urine output is maintained at a physiological minimum. Cerebral blood flow is maintained due to autoregulation but anxiety due to the circulating catecholamines is evident.
- **Class III**: 30–40% or 1500–2000 ml blood loss. The compensatory mechanisms are being exhausted and circulatory failure starts to develop. Tachycardia is marked and there is a measurable fall in systolic blood pressure. Tachypnoea is present due to reduced O_2 delivery to the tissues. Urine output decreases significantly, core-to-skin temperature difference increases further and mental changes are pronounced.
- **Class IV**: $\geq 40\%$ or ≥ 2000 ml blood loss results in circulatory failure, with compromised blood flow even to vital organs. Tachycardia is very high, systolic blood pressure markedly depressed, while diastolic pressure is still high; thus pulse pressure is very narrow. Urine output is negligible or zero, and if mean pressure falls below the autoregulatory level of the brain, the level of consciousness may be depressed. The skin feels cold because of vasoconstriction. Blood lactate, not shown in Figure 92, is significantly increased. Loss of $\geq 50\%$ or ≥ 2500 ml blood results in loss of consciousness and total circulatory failure.

Only some measurable physiological parameters are depicted in Figure 93; other changes such as skin colour and sweating are important in the evaluation of blood loss.

The response to haemorrhage described here is a typical one of a healthy individual. Heart disease, neuropathy or medication may produce a different response; some individuals respond with a paradoxical bradycardia.

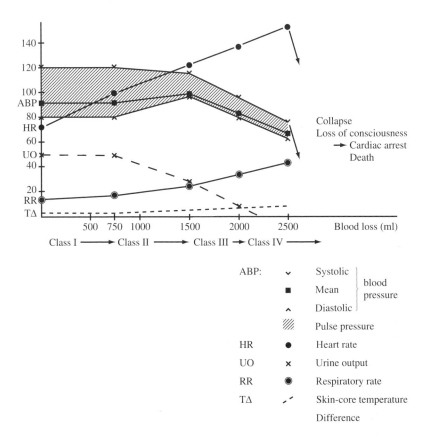

Figure 93. Changes in physiological parameters with blood loss (classes of haemorrhage).

Part 3a

Cerebral blood flow

Normal cerebral blood flow is 54 ml/100g/min (750 ml/min). The formula for flow indicates that flow is given by the ratio of pressure gradient (in this case cerebral perfusion pressure, which is the difference between mean arterial pressure and intracranial pressure), and resistance

$$Q = \Delta p / R = \frac{\text{MAP} - \text{ICP}}{R}. \tag{1}$$

Autoregulation exists to maintain, within physiological limits, a constant blood flow to the brain regardless of variations in arterial blood pressure and intracranial pressure; this is done by changes in cerebrovascular resistance, or by changing the perfusion pressure. As shown below, these factors are interrelated.

- **Mean arterial pressure**: Figure 94 shows how autoregulation maintains within physiological limits (normally 60–160 mmHg) constant cerebral blood flow. This is affected by changes in cerebral vascular resistance (see below). In chronic hypertension (or hypotension), the autoregulatory limits are moved up or down respectively. Outside the autoregulatory limits cerebral blood flow is pressure-dependent. When cerebral perfusion pressure is low due to high intracranial pressure (> 25–30 mmHg), baroreceptor stimulation produces systemic hypertension and cardioinhibitory centre stimulation produces reflex bradycardia (Cushing's reflex).
- **Intracranial pressure**: the relationship between intracranial fluid volume and pressure is shown in Figure 95 – **cerebral elastance** (or 'stiffness'), defined as $\Delta p / \Delta V$. Since the intracranial pressure is the dependent variable, it is logical to plot the pressure on the y-axis, and to use the term 'elastance' in this context. Elastance is the inverse of **cerebral compliance**, which is defined as $\Delta V / \Delta p$. In the graph elastance is given by the slope of the curve at any point, as shown. The skull is a rigid container filled with brain, cerebrospinal fluid and blood. As fluid is essentially incompressible, any increment in cerebral volume (e.g. in cerebral oedema) must be matched by a corresponding decrease of one of the other fluid components; cerebrospinal fluid can be to a certain extent pushed out of the foramen magnum, and venous blood is propelled out as the veins are compressed inside the skull. Since venous blood pressure is one of the components of intracranial pressure, a fall in the former (as venous blood is squeezed out) is accompanied by a fall in the latter. Thus, initially, a small increase in cerebral volume can be accommodated without a significant rise in intracranial pressure. When the compensatory limits are over stretched or lost, any small increment of cerebral volume (e.g. cough, drug or hypercarbia-induced vasodilatation) will be reflected in a steep rise in intracranial pressure, with a detrimental effect on cerebral blood flow.

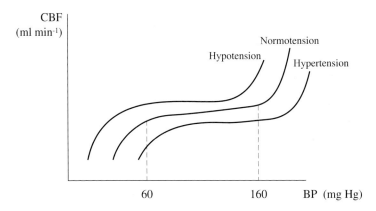

Figure 94. Cerebrovascular autoregulation.

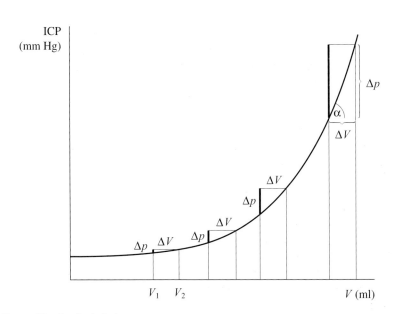

Figure 95. Cerebral elastance curve.

- **Cerebrovascular resistance**: the matching of cerebrovascular resistance to cerebral perfusion pressure is the basis of autoregulation of cerebral blood flow. The factors determining cerebrovascular resistance are:

1. **Partial pressure of CO_2**: cerebral arteriolar resistance is under the direct influence of local pCO_2 across a wide physiological range. Vasodilatation under normal intracranial pressure conditions results in a higher blood flow; this is partly the mechanism of autoregulation: if cerebral blood flow is reduced or if the cerebral metabolic rate is high, cerebral pCO_2 rises and pH falls, leading to vasodilatation and restoration of blood flow. In head injury, a mild degree of hypocapnia is preferable when ventilation is controlled under anaesthesia, provided blood pressure is maintained: intracranial pressure will fall as a result of venoconstriction and cerebral blood flow will improve. Very low levels of pCO_2 (< 3.4 kPa) lead to symptomatic cerebral ischaemia. Hypercapnia abolishes cerebrovascular autoregulation: cerebral blood flow is then directly proportional to mean arterial blood pressure, (as shown in Figure 96). Conversely, cerebrovascular response to CO_2 is blood pressure-dependent: in severe hypotension cerebral blood flow does not change with changes in CO_2 tension, as shown in Figure 97.

2. **Oxygen partial pressure** in the major cerebral arteries plays a role outside the physiological range; global cerebral blood flow only starts to rise when hypoxia is already significant. At the tissue level, however, O_2 partial pressure is probably the mechanism regulating local or regional blood flow in response to hypotension: reduced local blood flow with resulting tissue hypoxia produces immediate arteriolar vasodilatation. High levels of pO_2 are associated with a mild degree of vasoconstriction, i.e. reduced cerebral blood flow (as shown in Figure 97).

3. **Hydrogen ion concentration**: the effect is similar to, but independent of, pCO_2; the hydrogen ion is the mediator of flow metabolism coupling but it is not involved in the response to hypotension.

4. **Blood viscosity** influences vascular resistance as shown in the Hagen–Poiseuille formula (see above). The higher flow in haemodilution compensates (in part only) for otherwise reduced O_2 delivery due to the reduced haemoglobin concentration. This mechanism applies in cerebral circulation as in any other part of the body.

5. **Neurogenic and myogenic control**: apart from the humoral factors, the cerebrovascular tone is under sympathetic nervous control, and the autoregulation curve is shifted to the left or right according to the sympathetic tone. Myogenic response (increased tension in response to increased stretch) probably plays a part similar to other parts of the body.

In **head injury**, autoregulation is lost and the intracranial pressure may be elevated due to the presence of haematoma, cerebral oedema or both. Ventilation may be depressed with resulting hypercapnia: cerebral blood flow is then pressure-dependent. To prevent secondary brain injury, ventilation must be controlled and an adequate O_2 delivery to the brain ensured. A cerebral perfusion pressure > 60 mmHg is thought to provide adequate flow. From formula 1 it is then obvious that the desired mean arterial pressure must be kept at a level calculated as the sum of intracranial pressure + 60 mmHg.

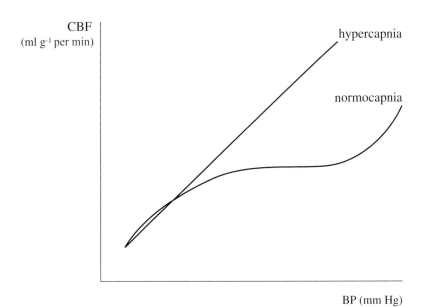

Figure 96. Autoregulation of cerebral blood flow within physiological limits; it is abolished by hypercapnia.

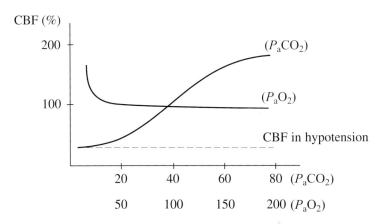

Figure 97. Cerebral blood flow as a function of arterial carbon dioxide tension (P_aCO_2) and oxygen tension (P_aO_2).

Coronary circulation

Myocardial blood flow is 200 ml/min, or 4% of cardiac output, for an organ weighing only 0.4% of body weight. Oxygen consumption of the heart is also high, 23 ml/min, or 9% of total. This is for a good reason: the heart is a pump that perfuses the rest of the body; its work is hard and it needs a constant energy supply from aerobic metabolism.

The coronary arteries are the first to receive oxygenated blood from the aorta; their **perfusion depends on the pressure gradient generated by the heart**. It is important to remember that coronary arteries run on the epicardial surface. The coronary arterial pressure gradient is thus from epicardium to endocardium, while the intramural pressure gradient during systole is in the opposite direction. Therefore, there is practically no endocardial flow during systole (see Figure 98 where coronary artery flow is plotted against the arterial pressure waveform) while the flow in epicardium is maintained. To compensate for the lack of perfusion in systole the subendocardial arteries are thought to be in a chronic state of dilation during diastole. At times of increased demand for perfusion, e.g. tachycardia, hypertension, this region is then unable to increase flow further and thus it is more susceptible to ischaemia.

Anaesthetic agents depress myocardial performance and oxygen consumption falls in line with reduced myocardial work (see Figure 100). Coronary blood flow therefore is reduced.

Myocardial ischaemia occurs when myocardial oxygen demand exceeds supply, i.e. when coronary blood flow and oxygen flow fall below the minimum required. In a diseased myocardium symptoms of ischaemia occur at a higher perfusion pressure, inside the lower limit of autoregulation. The prediction of cardiac events during anaesthesia is difficult but prevention should be practised: cardiac performance (power) is the product of mean arterial blood pressure and cardiac output. The output is the product of stroke volume and heart rate. Stroke volume is not easily assessed by bedside (or operating tableside) measurements but heart rate and blood pressure are monitored. Thus the **rate–pressure** product remains a useful clinical tool when estimating myocardial oxygen demand, and therapeutic manoeuvres can be directed at optimizing myocardial performance to maintain oxygen flow to the systemic circulation (which requires adequate cardiac output and haemoglobin concentration) while not overloading the heart by excessive pressures and rates.

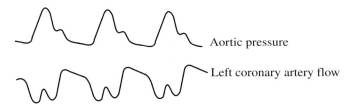

Aortic pressure

Left coronary artery flow

Figure 98. Coronary artery flow and arterial blood pressure.

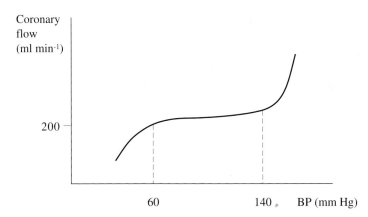

Figure 99. Coronary autoregulation.

3a

Autoregulation

Unlike the brain, which at times of need receives a higher perfusion pressure via baroreceptor stimulation, the heart cannot effectively increase its oxygen flow by increasing its perfusion pressure since the heart generates the pressure: myocardial oxygen consumption rises proportionately with myocardial work. The heart, therefore, regulates its perfusion only via changes in coronary artery resistance. The oxygen tension in the myocardium or a related parameter is the governing factor. Autoregulation maintains a constant blood flow in the coronary circulation within a wide range of pressures, 60–140 mmHg (see Figure 99). It must be kept in mind that the aortic diastolic pressure (not the mean arterial pressure) is the coronary perfusion pressure.

The sympathetic and parasympathetic nervous system affects the coronary vascular resistance, but this is modified by autoregulation: α-adrenergic stimulation produces coronary vasoconstriction but if coronary blood flow is compromised autoregulation results in vasodilatation. Parasympathetic stimulation, if unopposed, results in bradycardia. The accompanying fall in oxygen demand produces vasoconstriction; however, if a fast heart rate is maintained, vasodilatation prevails.

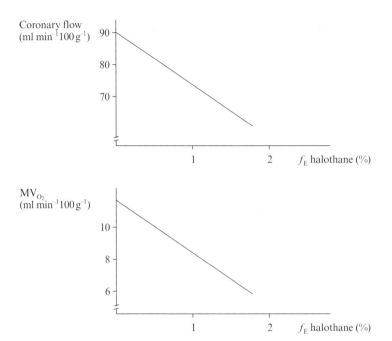

Figure 100. Effect of inhalational anaesthesia with halothane on coronary blood flow and myocardial oxygen consumption.

Part 3b

Physiology: the respiratory system

Oxyhaemoglobin dissociation curve

The oxyhaemoglobin dissociation curve (see Figure 101) describes oxygen binding to haemoglobin and its release in terms of haemoglobin saturation as a function of partial pressure oxygen. It is a sigmoid curve and it rather resembles the drug dose–effect relationship curve (see the chapter on pharmacology). However, in the case of the oxyhaemoglobin dissociation curve, the 'dose', i.e. oxygen partial pressure, is on a linear scale. This means that small, linear increments in oxygen partial pressure produce large changes in haemoglobin saturation on the straight part of the curve; at the extreme ends of the curve the opposite applies.

The central value on the straight part of the curve, which corresponds to haemoglobin saturation of 50%, is called the p_{50}; it is normally 3.6 kPa (26.6 mmHg). This is an unphysiological but convenient value to describe the position of the oxyhaemoglobin dissociation curve with respect to the pO_2. Points on the normal curve that correspond to the arterial and venous point are denoted as A and V. A shift of the oxyhaemoglobin dissociation curve to the right results in a higher p_{50}, and conversely a left shift lowers the p_{50}. The higher the p_{50}, the lower the affinity of haemoglobin for O_2.

Oxygen affinity (and therefore P_{50} in a reciprocal manner) is affected by the following interrelated factors:

- **2,3-Diphosphoglycerate** (2,3-DPG) concentration in the red cell: this is the primary control mechanism. 2,3-DPG is the allosteric effector that binds selectively to the deoxygenated haemoglobin, producing changes in haemoglobin molecule conformation. Oxygen affinity of haemoglobin is inversely related to 2,3-DPG concentration, therefore the oxyhaemo-globin dissociation curve is shifted to the right with a rise in 2,3-DPG.
- **[H$^+$]**: in this particular situation, [H$^+$] is preferable to pH since hydrogen ion concentration affects O_2 affinity in the same way as the other factors. A negative feedback mechanism through the effect of the hydrogen ion concentration on the 2,3-DPG concentration restores p_{50} back to normal.
- **pCO_2**: increasing the partial pressure of CO_2 increases p_{50}. This and the effect of pH was described by Bohr (Bohr effect). pH and pCO_2 are interrelated, but each is also a separate component.
- **Temperature**: There is also a negative feedback mechanism through the 2,3-DPG concentration.
- **Mean corpuscular haemoglobin concentration**: Mean corpuscular haemoglobin concentration changes rapidly with shifts in pH, to balance the slower changes in 2,3-DPG concentration.

For ease of O_2 delivery to the tissues, oxygen should bind easily to haemo-globin in the lung, and it should be easily released in the periphery.

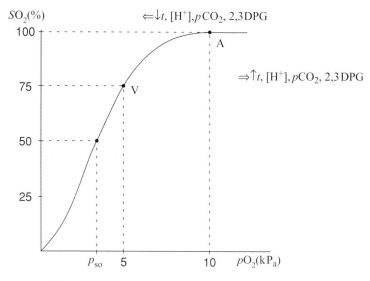

A arterial point at 96% saturation (10.7 kPa)

V venous point at 74% saturation (5.3 kPa)

Figure 101. Oxyhaemoglobin dissociation curve.

The body normally tends towards acidosis, constantly produces CO_2 and produces heat. These conditions result in a lower affinity of haemoglobin for O_2, to facilitate O_2 release in the tissues. The price for this is the necessary higher O_2 partial pressure that must be supplied. Conversely, to achieve adequate oxygen delivery, fetal haemoglobin must have a higher affinity than maternal haemoglobin for O_2. The fetal pH range is lower than maternal pH and this allows O_2 to be released in the fetal tissues.

Respiratory mechanics 1: Static properties, factors affecting compliance, closing volume

Elastic properties of the lungs and chest wall

From the mechanical point of view, the lungs are elastic sacs filled with air through tubes of varying resistance, attached on their outer surface to a container that is also elastic but which contains a rigid structure – the chest wall. Lung expansion has its limits; as the lungs are filled, pressure inside rises. The stiffer the lung, the higher the pressure rise will be for any given volume. **Compliance** is the reciprocal entity to stiffness, or elastance, and is defined as the change in volume over the change in pressure. It is the measure of the elastic properties of the lungs, chest wall or the total:

$$C = \Delta V / \Delta p \, (1 \text{ kPa}^{-1}).$$

Pulmonary pressures are usually measured in cmH_2O. Normal lung compliance would then be, for instance, 600 ml over 3 cmH_2O, or 200 ml.cmH_2O^{-1}.

Depending on where the pressure change is measured, compliance can be calculated for the lung, C_L (pressure difference measured from alveolus to pleural space), chest wall, C_{CW} (pressure difference measured from pleural space to atmosphere); the total, thoracic compliance C_T, is the sum of its components. When adding up compliance, it must be kept in mind that it is reciprocal to stiffness. Total stiffness is the sum of the individual components, while reciprocal values are added up for compliance.

$$1/C_T = 1/C_{CW} + 1/C_L$$
$$S_T = S_{CW} + S_L.$$

Under normal resting conditions, the retractive forces (elastic recoil) of the lung are balanced by the expansile forces of the chest wall; this balance governs the resting position. The elastic recoil of the lung draws it inwards; the resting position for the lung is at the end of expiration – the resting expiratory position. On the other hand, the elastic forces of the chest tend to expand it; the resting position for the chest wall is at the tidal volume level (500 ml higher than the resting position for the lung). In Figure 102a, the resting position of the isolated lung and isolated chest is shown for the right lung, and for the expanded lung on the left. The pressure gradients are shown for the resting expiratory position, and in the next drawing (Figure 102b) for the tidal breath position.

To expand the lung by 200 ml, a pressure difference of 1 cmH_2O has to be applied across the lung and 1 cmH_2O across the chest wall. Therefore the sum for total compliance would be:

$$C_T = \Delta V / \Delta p = 200/1 + 1 = 100 (\text{ml cmH}_2O^{-1}),$$

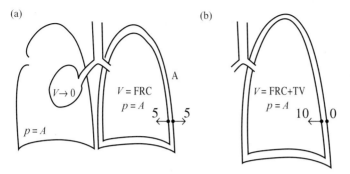

(a)   (b)

$V \rightarrow 0$

$p = A$

$V = FRC$
$p = A$

5   5

A

$V = FRC+TV$
$p = A$

10   0

Figure 102. Respiratory mechanisms. (a) resting position of the isolated lung and chest (right lung) and resting expiratory position of the normal lung at FRC (left lung). Atmospheric pressure $p = A$. Pressure gradients are shown as vectors, (b) pressure gradients after a tidal breath.

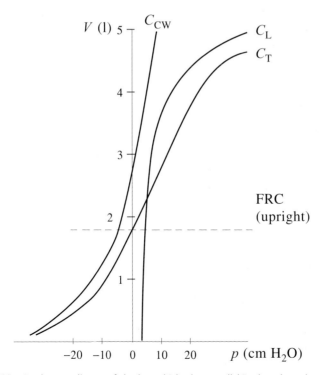

V (l)

C_{CW} C_L C_T

FRC
(upright)

p (cm H_2O)

Figure 103. Static compliance of the lung (C_L), chest wall (C_{CW}) and total compliance (C_T).

which means that total thoracic compliance is smaller than that each component. It is the stiffness of each that adds up directly. Therefore, to expand the
thorax by 500 ml, a pressure difference of 5 cm has to be applied.

The volume–pressure relationship of the lungs and chest wall are not
linear at the extremes of lung volume: at a high lung volume the lung opposes
further filling, i.e. its compliance is smaller (compliance slope less steep). In
Figure 103, the compliance is the slope of the line depicting the pressure-
volume relationship. At a low lung volume below the resting expiratory level,
the expansile force of the chest opposes further expiration, so that chest wall
compliance is smaller. This is reflected in the shape of each compliance curve.
Notice that the total compliance then becomes a sigmoid curve. The non-
linearity should be kept in mind when comparing different compliances: the
pressure difference for each value should be stated.

Factors affecting compliance are:

- **Disease**: in atelectasis, when the lung is relatively stiff, the point of
  balance (resting expiratory volume) will be reached at a lower lung
  volume, as there will be greater pull inwards; this will predispose to
  further atelectasis. The excessively compliant emphysematous lung has
  less elastic recoil; resting expiratory volume will then be greater, since the
  natural tendency for the chest wall to expand is maintained.
- **Age**: the immature lung in the infant is less elastic than in adulthood.
  Elasticity is highest in young adults and it decreases slowly with advancing
  age: lung compliance is therefore lowest in young adults. Chest wall
  compliance is highest at birth and slowly declines with age (see Figure
  104).
- **Posture**: thoracic compliance is lower in the supine position, as the
  gravitational pull of the abdomen, which existed in the upright position, is
  reversed and the diaphragm is pushed into the chest by the abdominal
  contents.
- **Anaesthesia**: several factors (supine position, airway closure, changes in
  intrathoracic blood volume, accumulation of fluid, direct effect of drugs,
  altered muscle tone, external pressure) influence compliance under
  anaesthesia; generally compliance is decreased.
- **Obesity**: the effect is compounded by supine or lithotomy position.

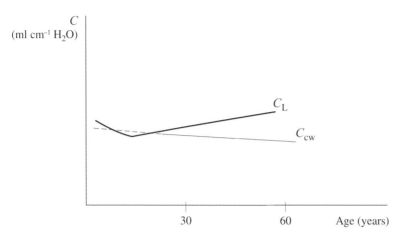

Figure 104. The effect of age on lung compliance (C_L) and chest wall compliance (C_{CW}).

Airways closure

Pleural pressure is influenced by the pressure of thoracic contents: it is less subatmospheric in the dependent lung zones then in the apex. When a normal subject exhales below the resting expiratory level, and towards the residual volume, pleural pressure eventually approaches or exceeds atmospheric pressure. The pressure gradient distending the small airways is thus lost, and the small airways will close; they will re-open only when a sufficient gradient is reached for their distension. The lung volume at which the airways close is called the **closing volume**. It increases more rapidly with age than the functional residual capacity. At around 65 years of age closing volume exceeds the FRC and airway closure occurs then during tidal breathing. The resulting **mismatching of ventilation and perfusion** is the explanation for the higher shunt fraction in the elderly. The relationship of closing volume and FRC is shown in Figure 105 for the upright and supine positions, and for the supine-anaesthetized patient. The further the closing volume line from the FRC line at a given age, the higher the shunt fraction. (See also the chapter on ventilation–perfusion relationship.)

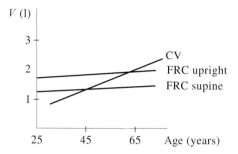

Figure 105. Changes in closing volume (CV) and functional residual capacity (FRC) during adulthood.

Respiratory mechanics 2: Dynamic properties, factors affecting resistance

Airway (non-elastic) resistance

Airway (non-elastic) resistance depends on the pattern of airflow (laminar or turbulent – see the relevant chapters), the rate of breathing and the radius and length of the airway, as described in the Hagen–Poiseuille formula. Remember that resistance is independent of flow in laminar flow but it rises linearly with flow in turbulent flow. Much higher pressures have to be achieved in turbulent flow to pass the same flow. (See also the chapter on flow for Reynolds number and the influence of viscosity and density.)

The radius decreases as the airways branch; the nasopharynx and larynx account for half of the total airway resistance, and the trachea and smaller airways constitute the other half. Airways smaller than 2 mm internal diameter contribute very little (see Figure 106). This is because their total cross-sectional area is large, and airflows in the small airways are lower, therefore laminar.

Factors affecting airway resistance are those which alter the diameter of the airway:

- **Body size**: the diameters of the larynx and trachea account for the large part of total resistance. Airway resistance is highest in neonates (30 cm l^{-1} per s) and declines with increasing body size until a functional residual capacity of 2500 is reached. Thereafter, the diameter of the airways and airways resistance does not change substantially as shown in Figure 107.
- **Thickness of bronchial mucosa**, e.g. swelling or secretions.
- **Bronchial muscle tone**: constriction due to parasympathetic stimuli, histamine release, irritant gases, dilatation produced by sympathetic stimuli or parasympathetic block.
- **Pressure gradients**: high-pressure gradient in atelectasis, etc. will distend airways, low-pressure gradient in emphysema results in smaller diameter of the airways.
- **Anaesthesia**: airway obstruction, effects of drugs.

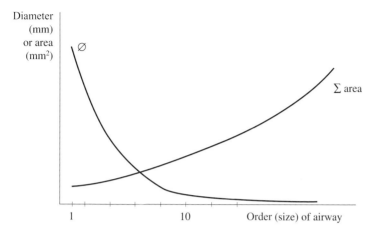

Figure 106. Size of airway and total cross-sectional area.

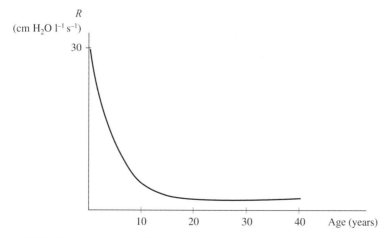

Figure 107. Airway resistance (R) and age.

Dynamic compliance

This is measured during normal tidal breathing. Figure 108 shows the plot of lung volumes and pressures for two sizes of breath in the normal lung, and a large breath in chronic obstructive airways disease. The slope of the axis of each loop is identical with the static compliance. It can be seen that for a normal (tidal) breath in the normal lung, the compliance slope is steeper than for a large breath, i.e. the lung is more compliant during normal tidal breathing than during a vital capacity breath. During a vital capacity breath in chronic obstructive airways disease, compliance slope is identical to the normal lung (or it could be higher if the disease progresses to emphysema) but the loop encompasses a greater area, indicating a greater work of breathing (see chapter on simple mechanics, work and power). This is understandable as the work is done against a higher airways resistance.

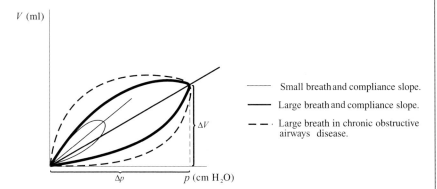

Figure 108. Dynamic compliance loops during spontaneous respiration.

Ventilation–perfusion relationship

Alveolar ventilation and its distribution

Approximately two-thirds of total ventilation reach the alveoli; one-third remains in the bronchi and is not available for gas exchange – **dead space gas**. Fresh gas that enters the alveoli per minute is known as **alveolar ventilation**; the normal value is about 5 l min^{-1}.

Alveolar ventilation is not distributed evenly in the lung: dependent regions are better ventilated during spontaneous respiration than the upper zones. This is because of the effects of gravity: pleural pressure at the base is less negative, and the alveoli at the base are less expanded than apical alveoli. In Figure 109, apical alveolus, represented by point A, is already nearly 80% expanded, while the basal alveolus at point B is only about 30% expanded. At maximum inspiration the change of size is higher for the basal alveoli than the apical ones, which had less scope for expansion. The above only applies for the normal lung at normal lung volumes. If basal alveoli are collapsed they receive no ventilation if the tidal breath, and the pleural pressure change is small. This is illustrated by point C (closed alveolus) in Figure 109. Such a situation occurs in the normal lung at residual volume, in old age when closing volume exceeds functional residual capacity or in chronic obstructive airways disease when functional residual capacity is high and the tidal breathing range is near the closing volume. Pleural pressure at the lung base exceeds atmospheric pressure in these situations, and a greater change in pressure gradient is required to re-expand basal alveoli, as shown.

Figure 110 illustrates how alveolar size changes across the lung from apex to base.

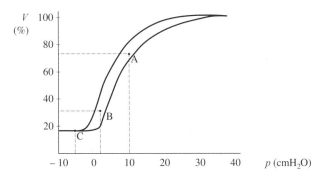

Figure 109. Lung pressure–volume diagram in a young, healthy adult.

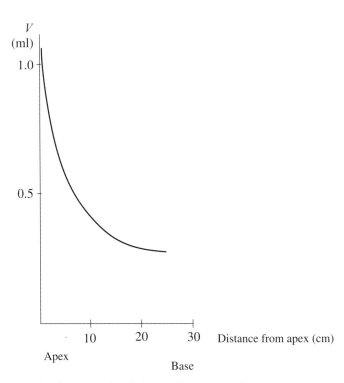

Figure 110. Alveolar volume in relation to distance from lung apex.

Pulmonary perfusion and its distribution

Blood flow distribution in the lung is also uneven, as the **arteriovenous pressure gradient**, which is a function of the **hydrostatic pressure** in the pulmonary arterial tree, is affected by **alveolar pressure**, which itself is a function of intrapleural pressure. The reduction in the arteriovenous pressure gradient (and therefore of flow) will be the greatest in the apex, where alveolar pressure is the highest; at the base, where alveolar pressure is low, the arteriovenous pressure gradient will be hardly affected by it. The result is that pulmonary blood flow is highest in the region where the ventilation is also highest – the base: this is the mechanism of **physiological ventilation–perfusion matching**.

The lung can be divided into three zones – the **West zones** – according to relative magnitude of the pulmonary arterial, venous and alveolar pressure. This is illustrated in Figure 111.

- In **zone 1** at the apex or non-dependent region, alveolar pressure may exceed the capillary pressure. The capillary then collapses and receives no flow. The ventilation that such an alveolus receives is dead space ventilation. In the normal lung, apical capillaries are just expanded; in hypotension or if alveolar pressure is artificially increased (e.g. in positive pressure ventilation), the **capillaries collapse** and give rise to **dead space effect**.
- In **zone 2** alveolar pressure is smaller than pulmonary arterial pressure but higher than the venous pressure. Here the **pressure gradient** for blood flow will be the **difference between arterial and alveolar pressure** (Starling resistor effect). Since the arterial pressure increases downward because of the hydrostatic effect, the pressure gradient and flow increase downwards too.
- In **zone 3** venous pressure exceeds alveolar pressure and all capillaries are held open. Blood **flow** is then the function of the **arteriovenous pressure gradient** as in other tissues.

At low lung volumes, blood flow to the base is reduced in the normal lung (thus matching reduced ventilation at the low volume) presumably because the basal blood vessels would be more compressed, rather than being held open wide as is the case at a normal lung volume. Another factor may be folds in pulmonary capillaries.

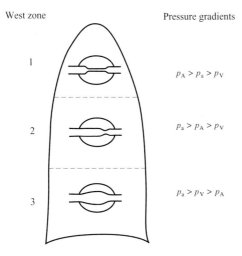

West zone

Pressure gradients

1

$p_A > p_a > p_V$

2

$p_a > p_A > p_V$

3

$p_a > p_V > p_A$

Figure 111. Diagram of the West zones of the lung.

Ventilation–perfusion ratio

Blood flow increases more rapidly with the distance from apex in the upright lung than ventilation. Blood flow at the base is 20 times higher than blood flow at apex, while basal ventilation is only three times higher than apical ventilation. As a consequence the ventilation/perfusion ratio (V/Q) diminishes from apex to base, to about 15% of the apical value at base. In other words, the apex is relatively over ventilated while the base is relatively over perfused. This is the basis of the physiological **ventilation/perfusion inequality**. Figure 112 illustrates this schematically. Ventilation of unperfused alveoli at the apex contributes to the **physiological dead space effect**, as mentioned above: inhaled fresh gas is wasted and is unavailable for gas exchange. Perfusion of unventilated alveoli at the base means that blood flowing through this region will receive no oxygen, and will contribute to the **physiological shunt**. In the normal lung the base receives most of the pulmonary blood flow; as the blood there is less well oxygenated, the result is a venous admixture, normally up to 5%. Well ventilated but **under perfused apical regions cannot compensate for the shunt** by increasing oxygenation of the blood that they receive, as the blood is already fully saturated with oxygen; this is due to the shape of oxygen dissociation curve. Carbon dioxide exchange, however, is a linear function of its partial pressure; apical alveoli can compensate to a large extent for the excess CO_2 arising from the non-ventilated basal alveoli. Thus end-tidal (alveolar) to arterial gradient for CO_2 is < 1 mmHg, or 0.13 kPa, while the end-tidal to arterial gradient for O_2 is several mmHg. Increased total ventilation of a normal lung can compensate for both, as the basal well-perfused alveoli will then receive more ventilation.

During **anaesthesia** changes in dead space and shunt fraction occur: as shown previously, closing volume is above functional residual capacity in most anaesthetized patents. Endobronchial intubation increases the shunt fraction substantially (one lung perfused but not ventilated). A higher inspired oxygen concentration can only partly compensate for this. Dead space changes follow changes in cardiac output, e.g. hypotension.

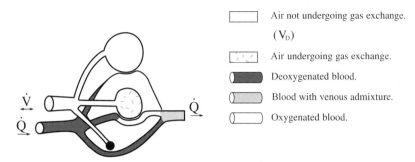

Air not undergoing gas exchange.
(V_D)

Air undergoing gas exchange.

Deoxygenated blood.

Blood with venous admixture.

Oxygenated blood.

Figure 112. Schematic drawing of ventilation–perfusion relationship in the three zones of the lung.

Oxygen cascade, oxygen therapy and shunt fraction

Oxygen cascade

The oxygen cascade depicted in Figure 113 shows the decrease in oxygen tension at each stage of oxygen transport from the ambient air into the tissue.

Notice that **alveolar oxygen tension**, $P_AO_2 = 13.3$ kPa, is substantially lower than oxygen tension in ambient air. This is because alveolar gas has a different composition from ambient air: inhaled air is fully saturated with water vapour on inspiration and it then mixes in the alveoli with gas that already underwent gas exchange.

Alveolar oxygen tension can be calculated from the Nunn equation (see the chapter on Gas R line for more details).

The **arterial–alveolar tension gradient** will depend on the diffusing capacity of the alveolar membrane, cardiac output, rate of binding of oxygen with haemoglobin (these are the factors affecting **gas transfer**) and on shunt fraction. In the normal lung, and with the other conditions being normal, the most important factor is the **physiological shunt**.

Oxygen tension in the **capillary** is further reduced as a result of the uptake by the tissues. If oxygen extraction is poor (for instance, in low cardiac output states when oxygen delivery does not match oxygen demand, or in mitochondrial poisoning), capillary and venous oxygen tension is relatively high while the tissues suffer hypoxia.

Each step of oxygen transport down the cascade can be altered by abnormal conditions or pathological changes. To achieve the target mitochondrial oxygen tension of 0.13–1.3 kPa, inspired oxygen tension must be raised to increase the pressure gradient if such abnormal conditions exist. In the case of mitochondrial poisoning, this is very difficult as only the unaffected mitochondria utilize the oxygen supplied. The oxygen pressure gradient has to be increased to 100%; even so, the extent of tissue hypoxia will depend on the degree of poisoning. At the other end of oxygen cascade it is possible to lower inspired oxygen concentration in the ambient air without significantly affecting oxygen supply (this is the basis of expired air mouth-to-mouth resuscitation). It can be seen that the further down the oxygen cascade, the higher the inspired oxygen tension must be to compensate for a lesion that makes the gradient steeper.

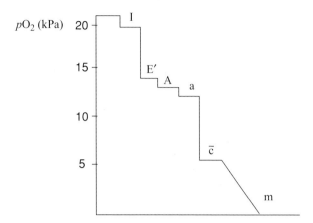

I = inspired (warmed humidified) air.
E′ = end-expiratory gas.
A = ideal alveolar gas.
a = arterial blood.
c̄ = mean capilary blood.
m = mitochondria.

Figure 113. The oxygen cascade.

Iso shunt lines

Iso shunt lines shown in Figure 114 illustrate the effect of increasing the inspired oxygen tension on arterial oxygen tension, for various shunt fractions. Assumptions are made about the other variables affecting oxygen delivery (normal haemoglobin, normal oxygen extraction, normal arterial pH and CO_2 tension, normal gas transfer). Inspired oxygen tension (f_1O_2) is the controlled parameter, and arterial oxygen tension (p_aO_2) is its function. Zero shunt is included although it only exists in theory: there is a linear relationship between f_1O_2 and p_aO_2. Physiological shunt of up to 5% and pathological shunt of up to 10% are highly responsive to oxygen therapy: the slope of linear relationship is steep with the exception of the lower end of the line, and the line is parallel to the zero shunt line. Between an f_1O_2 of 0.21 and about 0.35 for 5% shunt, or 0.45 for 10% shunt, the slope is less steep (less increment of arterial pO_2 with increased f_1O_2). With increasing shunt fractions the slope is reduced up to progressively higher inspired oxygen concentrations. A 50% shunt is hardly affected by increasing the f_1O_2 at all; arterial pO_2 stays low even when breathing pure oxygen. Therapeutic efforts in this case must be directed towards removing the cause of the shunt.

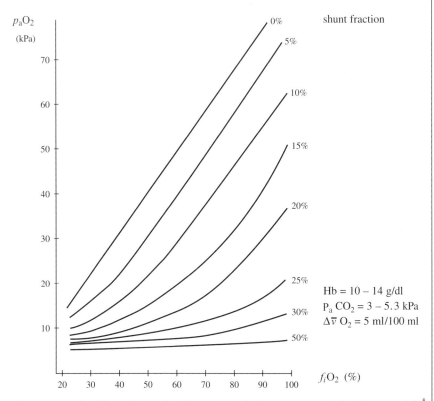

Figure 114. The effect of shunt function and inspired oxygen fraction (f_iO_2) on arterial oxygen (p_aO_2). Assumptions as above are made.

Gas R line, solution of the ventilation/perfusion model

The gas R line is the O_2/CO_2 diagram shown in Figure 115. It depicts the relationship between **lung volumes** and the **partial pressures of the respiratory gases**. It shows how the anatomical and physiological dead space influence the partial pressure of CO_2, and how the magnitude of alveolar ventilation and partial pressure of inspired O_2 affect alveolar partial pressure of O_2.

The volumes in the diagram are shown on the R line:

$$V_{Dalv} = \text{alveolar dead space (points A–É),}$$
$$V_{Danat} = \text{anatomical dead space (points É–Ē),}$$
$$V_{Dphys} = \text{physiological dead space (points A–È),}$$
$$V_A = \text{ideal alveolar ventilation (points Ē–I),}$$
$$V_E = \text{ventilatory volume measured during expiration (points A–I).}$$

Point A denotes alveolar; point I denotes inspired.
The partial pressures are in the following gases:

$$p_a = \text{arterial gas}$$
$$p_{É} = \text{end-tidal gas}$$
$$p_{Ē} = \text{mixed expired gas}$$
$$p_i = \text{inspired gas.}$$

An assumption is made that

$$p_{aCO_2} = p_{ACO_2} \text{ (arterial } p_{CO_2} = \text{alveolar } p_{CO_2}).$$

Partial pressures of CO_2 are plotted on the vertical axis, and partial pressures of O_2 on the horizontal axis. The distance between various points on the R line corresponds to the lung volumes shown.

The basis of the graph is the fact that gas exchange for O_2 and CO_2 occurs in opposite directions: inspired gas contains a higher concentration of O_2 and no CO_2; after gas exchange, the concentration of O_2 in the expired gas is lower than that in inspired gas while the concentration of CO_2 increased from zero to the end-tidal value.

The **gas equations** have been derived from this plot. The coordinates of the various points on the R line, the axes, and the R line itself form right-angled triangles; according to the laws of geometry the ratios of any pair of similar sides are equal. Therefore

$$V_{Dphys}/V_E = A\bar{E}/AI = p_{aCO_2} - p_{ECO_2}/p_aCO_2 \text{ (the Bohr equation),}$$

or, in other words, the ratio of dead space ventilation to total ventilation is the same as the ratio of the difference between partial pressures of CO_2 in arterial

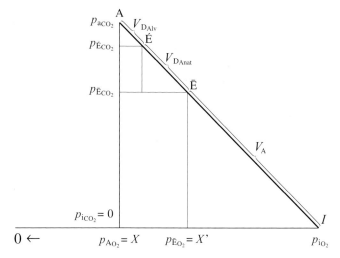

Figure 115. Gas R line.

blood and the expired gas to arterial p_{CO_2}. Another variant of this equation is:

$$V_{Dalv}/V_E = A\acute{E}/AI = p_{aCO_2} - p_{\bar{E}CO_2}/p_{aCO_2},$$

or, in other words, the ratio of alveolar dead space to total ventilation is the same as the ratio of the arterial end-tidal pressure gradient for CO_2 to arterial p_{CO_2}. The nominator in the equation, the **arterial to end-tidal pressure gradient for CO_2**, is easily measured and serves to assess the **magnitude of dead space**.

The ideal alveolar oxygen tension is calculated from the **Nunn equation**. Notice that point X is not zero as alveolar p_{O2} is not zero; therefore p_{AO2} has to be subtracted from the values on the horizontal axis:

$$IX/IX' = AI/\bar{E}I,$$

therefore

$$p_{iO_2} - p_{AO_2}/p_{iO_2} - p_{\bar{E}O_2} = p_{aCO_2}/p_{\bar{E}O_2}.$$

All gas tensions, except p_{AO2}, can be measured. Then

$$p_{AO_2} = p_{iO_2} - p_{\hat{a}CO_2}(p_{iO_2} = p_{\bar{E}O_2}/p_{\bar{E}CO_2}),$$

where p_{iO_2} and $p_{\bar{E}O_2}$ are measured directly by the paramagnetic oxygen analyser (or any of the other oxygen analysis methods), p_{aCO_2} is measured directly from arterial blood sample and $p_{\bar{E}CO_2}$ is measured in expired gas collected into a Douglas bag, with an infrared CO_2 analyser.

The Nunn equation is used for the calculation of the alveolar p_{O_2}, which is then used in the calculation of the **shunt fraction**, not derived here.

$$Q_s/Q_t = c_c - c_a/c_c - c_{\bar{v}},$$

where c is oxygen content, and the subscripts are c for end-pulmonary capillary, a for arterial and $\bar{v}$ more mixed venous blood. Arterial and mixed venous oxygen content is measured directly by the Van Slyke method or any of the other oxygen analysis methods; mixed venous blood is sampled from the pulmonary artery catheter. End-pulmonary capillary blood cannot be sampled but oxygen tension in the pulmonary capillary is assumed to be in equilibrium with alveolar oxygen tension, derived from the Nunn equation. Oxygen content in the pulmonary capillary is then calculated from the saturation, assuming a normal oxyhaemoglobin dissociation curve.

Hypoxia is a powerful respiratory stimulus. In figure 116, pulmonary ventilation in litres per minute is plotted against arterial oxygen tension in kilopascals (thick line). The horizontal axis is truncated above 17 kPa and shows extrapolation at abnormally high levels of hyperoxia.

It can be seen that the curve has a shape similar to a rectangular hyperbola, whereby the minute ventilation stays almost the same above 12 kPa of arterial oxygen tension but starts rapidly increasing when arterial pO_2 is reduced below this level. From the chapter on mathematical concepts in Part 1 we know that a rectangular hyperbola describes a **reciprocal relationship**, in this case between **arterial pO_2 and minute ventilation**. Hypoxia below 7 kPa produces a steep rise in minute ventilation, theoretically *ad infinitum*. Notice that the vertical asymptote is at 4 kPa, as oxygen tension below this level becomes incompatible with life. The horizontal asymptote is at a level slightly below normal minute ventilation (although in this particular case the 'normal' level is somewhat high at almost 10 litres per minute).

The thin line in the graph represents the relationship between **arterial oxygen saturation and minute ventilation**. This is an approximately **linear relationship** with a negative gradient. Notice that the horizontal axis for arterial oxygen saturation is only shown for values between 70% and 90%, as the relationship between these two parameters is roughly linear within these limits (see oxyhaemoglobin dissociation curve, page 131). Ventilatory response to oxygen below arterial oxygen saturation of 70% has not been tested in humans.

There is a high individual variability in the hypoxic response, which explains poor adaptation of some individuals to high altitude.

The hypoxic response is augmented by hypercapnia: small increases of arterial carbon dioxide move the threshold of hypoxic response (curve shifted to the right) and increase the slope of the curve.

Anaesthetic drugs reduce the hypoxic ventilatory drive, even at sub anaesthetic doses. This is only one of the reasons why anaesthetised patients and patients recovering from an anaesthetic are given an oxygen enriched gas mixture, usually above 30%. The hypoxic ventilatory drive is also reduced during natural sleep, explaining reduced oxygen saturations during sleep. In patients with obstructive sleep apnoea, this response is so diminished that the patients intermittently become apnoeic, and only profound hypoxia as a result of the apnoea provides a sufficient stimulus for the respiration to resume.

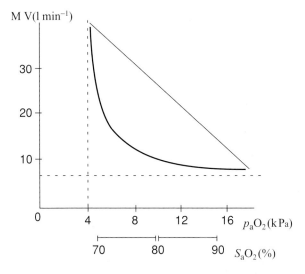

Figure 116. Ventilatory response to oxygen.

Ventilatory response to carbon dioxide

Carbon dioxide, up to an arterial tension of about 15 kPa in normal subjects, is a respiratory stimulant. In figure 117, pulmonary minute volume as percentage of normal is plotted against arterial pCO$_2$. Pulmonary minute volume increases in an approximately linear fashion up to 15 kPa. The response decreases sharply above 15 kPa and the slope has a reverse gradient after 20 kPa.

Beyond 20 kPa, hypercapnia becomes irreversible because of the vicious spiral of reduced minute ventilation leading to a further rise in P_aCO$_2$, leading to a further reduction in minute volume. Simply removing the original cause of hypercapnia, for instance rebreathing from an anaesthetic circuit, will not reverse this course – it is necessary to start artificial ventilation to remove the excess carbon dioxide.

Only the straight portion of the ascending limb has been determined in humans. Minute ventilation below normocapnia is reduced and the line is extrapolated to zero at both ends.

Normal responsiveness of the respiratory centre to carbon dioxide is on average 15 litre. min^{-1} kPa^{-1} (2 litre min^{-1} per mmHg).

In patients with chronic obstructive airways disease, the curve is shifted to the right, so that minute ventilation is low at carbon dioxide levels which would be stimulant in normal subjects. It is useful to know the 'normal' level for a patient with chronic lung disease before commencing artificial ventilation, in order not to hyperventilate when discontinuing the artificial ventilation. Because of their decreased sensitivity to carbon dioxide, hypoxia becomes the predominant stimulus in patients with type II respiratory failure, and oxygen therapy needs to be controlled in this situation.

Conversely, ventilatory response to carbon dioxide is increased in pregnant women and the curve is shifted to the left.

Carbon dioxide was used as a respiratory stimulant during induction of anaesthesia when the intended mode of ventilation was spontaneous respiration. It was added in a concentration of 5% to the inspired gas mixture; the advantage of this method was that manual hyperventilation could be used to ensure fast uptake of the inhalational agent, without causing hypocapnia and respiratory depression. Unfortunately, accidents with carbon dioxide flowmeter being left open at full flow resulted in carbon dioxide narcosis and therefore this practice is no longer encouraged. Carbon dioxide cylinders must not be left on an anaesthetic machine, and modem machines do not have the CO$_2$ yoke. Circle systems allow taking the absorber out of circuit, and this also produces hypercapnia and respiratory stimulation.

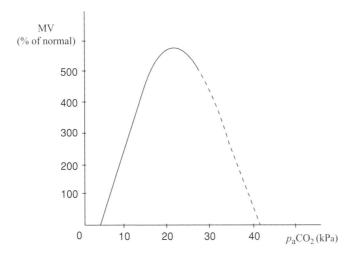

Figure 117. Approximate shape of carbon dioxide response curve.

Part 4

Pharmacology

Drug elimination

Drug elimination, like other natural processes of elimination, is in many instances an exponential decay process (see the chapter on exponentials for more details and graphs). The **elimination constant**, k, of this process is directly proportional to clearance of the drug's and indirectly proportional to the volume of distribution. The time constant is inverted elimination rate constant. Therefore

$$k = Cl/V_D$$
$$\tau = 1/k = V_D/Cl.$$

The concentration of the drug in the body at any time can then be calculated from the basic exponential decay equation.

$$C = C_o e^{-t/\tau} = C_o e^{-kt} = C_o.e^{-t \cdot Cl/V}.$$

First- and zero-order kinetics

From the properties of the exponential decay curve it is known that the rate of decay at any time is proportional to the ordinate at that point; applied to drug elimination this means that **rate of elimination** is **dependent on the drug concentration** at the chosen time point. Mathematically denoted this would be:

$$dc/dt = -kc^1,$$

where k = elimination rate constant, which is characteristic for each drug. Figure 118 of the drug illustrates the **first-order kinetics** formula: the higher the concentration, the higher the rate of change in concentration. The slope of the relationship between drug concentration and its rate of elimination is the value of the elimination rate constant. Remifentanil, which is cleared fast, has a steep slope (high elimination rate constant). Alfentanil, which is cleared more slowly, has a gentle slope.

By contrast, the relationship of alcohol elimination to alcohol concentration has two phases, the first phase being **zero-order kinetics**. Note that in the equation above, concentration is raised (mathematically quite unnecessarily) to the power of 1; it would have sufficed just to write c. The power of 1 relates to the term first-order kinetics. In zero-order kinetics, when the physiological processes of drug elimination are overwhelmed (enzymes saturated), the **rate of drug elimination** is independent of drug concentration and **depends on the elimination rate constant only**. In Figure 119 the rate of alcohol elimination is constant during the initial phase, conforming to the formula

$$dc/dt = -kc^o = -k.$$

When blood alcohol is < 0.05 mg ml^{-1}, first-order kinetics apply.

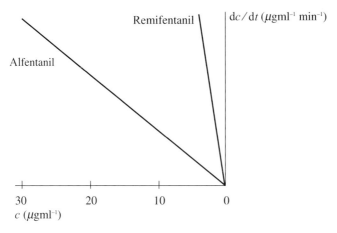

Figure 118. First-order kinetics of remifentanil and alfentanil.

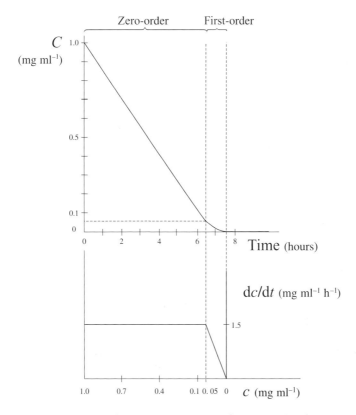

Figure 119. Zero-order and first-order elimination of blood alcohol from 1 mg^{-1} to complete elimination.

First-order kinetics are also called linear pharmacokinetics, because the **rate** of drug elimination has a linear relationship to the drug concentration. However, drug concentration as a function of time falls exponentially! The exponential decay curve can be transformed into a straight line when drug concentration is plotted on a logarithmic scale (see the chapter Exponentials 1). Drug elimination half-life can then be easily read off this plot.

Compartmental models

So far, the pharmacokinetic model assumed that the drug, after intravenous injection, was rapidly and uniformly distributed throughout the body, and then rapidly excreted. This is called the **one-compartment model**, i.e. the body behaves as one pharmacokinetic compartment. An example that can be applied to this situation is an injection of suxamethonium.

For most drugs, however, their tissue concentration depends not only on the plasma concentration but also on their lipid solubility and protein binding. Tissue concentration in richly perfused organs approaches that in plasma; these form a **small central compartment**. The rest of the body then form a **larger peripheral compartment**, which slowly achieves equilibrium with the central compartment, depending on drug transfer constants between the compartments. This **two-compartment model** approximates reality better than the single-compartment model.

Drug concentration in the central compartment (plasma) will then follow a more complicated pattern than that of a single exponential decay; the drug can leave the central compartment by either transfer (distribution) to the peripheral compartment or by elimination from the body. Initially, when drug concentration is high in the central compartment but low in the peripheral compartment, the drug leaves the central compartment chiefly by distribution to the peripheral compartment. This is **the distribution or α phase**, with its own transfer constant, k_α, and distribution half-life, $t_{1/2\alpha}$.

When the peripheral compartment concentration equilibrated with that in the central compartment, the drug then leaves the compartment by the process of elimination from the body. This is the final **elimination phase β**, with its elimination rate constant, k_β, and elimination (or terminal) half-life, $t_{1/2\beta}$. Drug elimination can then be described by the biexponential equation:

$$C = C_1 e^{-\alpha t} + C_2 e^{-\beta t},$$

where C_1 = initial drug concentration at time $t = 0$, and C_2 = theoretical drug concentration at time $t = 0$ if the elimination phase had applied to the whole process. α and β denote the elimination rate constants in this formula. In Figure 120 C_2 is the intercept of the extrapolated slope of the elimination phase with the ordinate. Notice that the plot is semi-logarithmic; during the transitional phase the line is curved as the two processes (distribution and elimination) happen simultaneously.

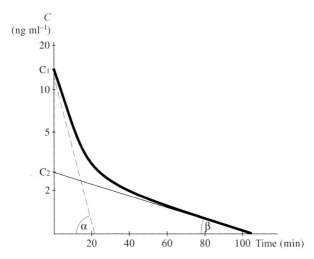

Figure 120. Biexponential decline in plasma concentration of a drug after intravenous injection in a two-compartment model.

Uptake and distribution of inhalational anaesthetic agents

This chapter deals only with uptake in high gas flow. The following formula describes the **factors** involved in the uptake of inhalational anaesthetic agents:

$$f_{A\,an} = f_{i\,an} - \dot{V}_{an}/\dot{V}_A,$$

where $f_{A\,an}$, $f_{i\,an} =$ **alveolar and fractional inspired concentration of the agent**, respectively, $V_{an} =$ **uptake** of the agent and $V_A =$ **alveolar ventilation**.

In other words, alveolar concentration depends on how much is 'put in' ($f_{i\,an}$) and 'taken out' (V_{an}/V_A).

The rate of rise of f_{Aan} as a function of time can also be plotted as the rate of rise of the fraction f_A/f_i. This merely describes alveolar concentration as a fraction of the inspired concentration. From the equation above, it follows that

$$f_A/f_i = 1 - \dot{V}_{an}/\dot{V}_A f_i,$$

It can be seen from this equation that alveolar concentration as a fraction of inspired concentration (f_A/f_i) will be approaching 1 (the desired aim of swift induction) when the fraction $\dot{V}_{an}/\dot{V}_A f_i$ is small or negligible. The bigger the factors in the denominator ($\dot{V}_A$, f_i), the smaller the fraction. In other words, high alveolar ventilation and high fractional-inspired concentration of the anaesthetic increase the rate of rise of alveolar concentration. The reverse is true of the factors that enhance the uptake of the inhalational agent namely cardiac output, shunt fraction and blood solubility of the agent.

The **rate of rise of alveolar concentration** can then be plotted as shown in Figure 121; the factors mentioned above influence it in the predicted manner: an upward shift of the curve occurs with increased alveolar ventilation, increased inspired concentration, reduced cardiac output, reduced shunt fraction, lower blood solubility and vice versa. The time axis on the top diagram has no markings as this is an idealised representation; the markings would be different for each inhalational agent, depending on their blood solubility.

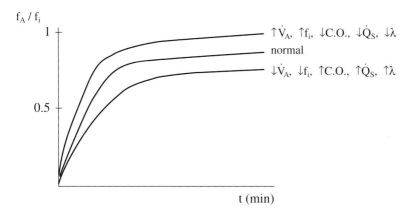

Figure 121. Factors influencing alveolar gas or vapour concentration during uptake.

The effect of blood solubility of an agent on the rate of uptake is shown in Figure 122. Sevoflurane has the lowest blood solubility and is taken up almost as rapidly as nitrous oxide, with the f_A to f_i ratio greater than 50% in about 2 minutes. The rate of washout on discontinuation of the agent would be similarly rapid.

Interaction occurs among the factors above: changes in alveolar ventilation and/or cardiac output affect most those anaesthetic agents with high blood solubility. With agents such as nitrous oxide, where the rate of rise of alveolar concentration is fast, the effect of changes in alveolar ventilation and/or cardiac output is negligible.

The premise that the partial pressure of the anaesthetic in the brain (and therefore the speed of induction) closely follows the anaesthetic partial pressure in the alveoli only holds for normal cerebral perfusion. Thus the effects of altered minute ventilation or cardiac output on the speed of inhalational induction may be modified by the effect of these factors on cerebral vasculature. Cerebral vasoconstriction caused by hyperventilation could in theory slow down the rate of induction (instead of increasing it). Similarly, in decompensated shock there may be a reduction in cerebral blood flow, which may offset a theoretical rapid induction.

In practice, however, this is rarely observed: during inhalational induction, patients usually breathe from a semi-closed rebreathing circuit. The rise in arterial pCO_2 as a result of rebreathing would mostly offset the effects on the cerebral perfusion mentioned above during hyperventilation. As regards decompensated shock, in this situation inhalational agents are used with great caution, in doses that would be subanaesthetic in haemodynamically stable patients, because of myocardial depression and the already altered state of consciousness. Swift inhalational induction aided by high inspired concentration of the inhalation agent is not the aim here – maintenance of mean arterial pressure and cerebral perfusion pressure take precedence. The theoretical principles considered here are useful to keep in mind, but do not forget the wider picture.

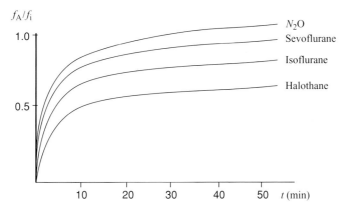

Figure 122. Rate of rise of alveolar concentration for different anaesthetic agents.

Pharmacodynamic effects of drugs

Most but not all drugs produce their effects by binding to receptor sites. When an active drug binds to its receptor site, the receptor changes its configuration to its active state, and this initiates an intracellular response in the effector tissue, and eventually results in the drug's effect.

This binding is reversible, with an equilibrium that depends on the association and dissociation constants of the process.

$$\text{Drug} + \text{receptor} \overset{k_1}{\underset{k_2}{\leftrightarrows}} \text{drug} - \text{receptor complex} \rightarrow \text{effect.}$$

Dose–response curve

The dose–response curve is the plot of the dose of a drug against its effect, usually expressed as the percentage of maximum effect. Initially, the effect rises steeply up to 50%; thereafter, progress to the maximum effect is slower, with much higher doses required to produce the ceiling effect. The graphical result is a **rectangular hyperbola** (Figure 123), conforming to the formula

$$y = a - 1/x.$$

If the graph is re-plotted with log dose on the ordinate, the result is a **sigmoid shape**. This has advantages: it allows a greater range of doses to be represented, and it allows easy comparison of drug dosages on the straight part of the curve by the means of comparing their efficacy and potency. To produce an effect, a drug has to bind to the receptor site; its affinity for the receptor therefore affects both its efficacy and its potency. These terms are explained below.

Affinity

Affinity is a measure of the ability of a drug to bind to the receptor site and form a stable complex. Pure **agonist** drugs have a high affinity for the **active state** of the receptor, whereas pure **antagonists** have a high affinity for its **inactive state**. Thus, drugs with a high affinity for the same receptor can have very different effects, depending on their intrinsic activity, or efficacy (see below). Affinity may be expressed by an IC_{50}, which is the concentration producing 50% inhibition of the binding of a highly selective ligand. Among agonist drugs, there is a high correlation between their IC_{50} and their potency. The relationship between affinity and efficacy is not only complicated by the degree of agonism, as mentioned above, but also by other limiting factors that may be involved in the process of the biological response, e.g. the presence of other ligands, second messengers, etc. A well-known example is the degree of acetylcholine receptor occupancy by non-depolarizing relaxants versus the degree of neuromuscular block.

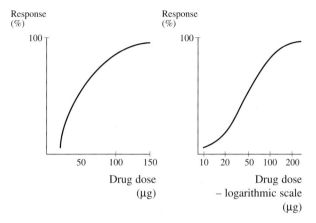

Figure 123. Drug dose and effect.

Efficacy (intrinsic activity)

The maximum effect that a drug is capable of producing is its efficacy, i.e. it is the **plateau of the dose–response curve**; in other words, efficacy indicates the limit of the dose–response relationship on the y (effect)-axis.

Pure **agonists** have a high affinity for the active state of the receptor site (e.g. morphine and the μ receptor), and are **100% efficacious**. **Antagonist** drugs (e.g. naloxone and the μ receptor) have no intrinsic activity (they have a high affinity for the inactive state of the receptor site), and are **not effi-cacious**. **Partial agonists** (e.g. nalorphine and the μ receptor, β-adrenergic blockers with intrinsic sympathomimetic activity and the β-adrenergic recep-tor) have only low affinity for the active receptor site, so that even at maximum receptor occupancy not all receptor sites will be activated. Therefore, partial agonists have a lower intrinsic activity or **efficacy < 100%**. Full and partial agonist opioid log dose–response curves are shown in Figure 124; the plot for naloxone is identical with the x-axis. Buprenorphine and nalorphine have not only lower affinity than fentanyl but also a lower efficacy than all three full agonists – they do not achieve 100% response.

Potency

The potency of a drug is a measure of the **mass of the drug** required to produce a certain **level of effect**. Clearly it is not useful to chose 100% effect as the dose–response relationship is lost at that level. A **reference point** on the dose–response curve is therefore chosen to allow a comparison, usually **50% of the maximum effect**. A drug that produces the same (50%) effect with only 1/10th of the dose (mass) of another drug is 10 times more potent (e.g. pethidine and morphine). Relative potency of morphine versus pethidine is therefore 10, calculated as the ratio of equipotent doses. Potency can be illustrated as the **position** of the log dose–response curve **along the x** (dose)-axis; the less potent a drug, the further its dose–response curve lies along the x-axis (Figure 124).

Antagonism

Competitive antagonists

Competitive antagonists **occupy reversibly** some of the available **receptor sites**; if a higher dose of active drug is given, it can still achieve its maximum effect. Competitive agonists, therefore, **in effect reduce the potency** of a drug, but **not its efficacy** (the dose–response curve shifts along the x-axis, the shape is unchanged). Naloxone reversibly antagonizes opioid drugs; in its presence the log dose–response curves are shifted to the right, as shown opposite on the example of pethidine.

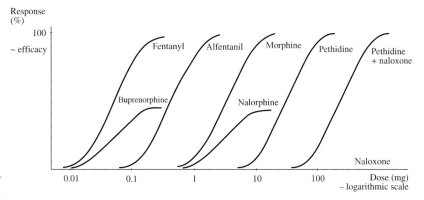

Figure 124. Opioid drugs log dose–response curves.

Non-competitive antagonists

Non-competitive antagonists bind **irreversibly** to the receptor sites; thus they make some (or all) of the receptor sites unavailable to the active drug. Increasing the dose of the active drug does not achieve a full effect. Non-competitive antagonists thus **reduce the efficacy** of a drug, while its **potency**, at least in the lower part of the curve, is **relatively unchanged**. The picture produced is the same as that of partial agonist drugs. In Figure 125, compare the log dose–response curve of norepinephrine under normal conditions, in the presence of a competitive blocker (phentolamine) and in non-competitive antagonism by increasing doses of phenoxybenzamine.

To quantify the degree of partial agonism by various agonists, pA_2 has been devised. This is the negative logarithm of the concentration of the antagonist necessary to produce a particular level of response. Thus, pure agonists at one type of opioid receptor, such as μ (morphine, β-endorphine) have the same pA_2 for naloxone (7), while pA_2 for leu-enkephalin is about 6. In other words, ten times more naloxone is needed to antagonise the effects of leu-enkephalin than to antagonize β-endorphine. (Remember that a difference of 1 unit on the logarithmic scale is ten times the difference on the linear scale.) This suggests that these two agents act on different receptor populations, an observation which was postulated even before the δ receptor (at which leu-enkephalin is an agonist) was isolated.

Therapeutic index

The therapeutic index is a measure of the safety of a drug in clinical use. **Reference points** on two integrated probability curves (otherwise known as centile curves) need be compared; one for a desired clinical effect, the other for a toxic effect. The centile curve resembles the log dose–response curve but is different: the y-axis represents the percentage of population that responds at the given dose; the x-axis scale is linear, as shown in Figure 126. The reference point is a dose that produces the chosen effect in 50% of the individuals. ED_{50} is the median effective dose (which produces the clinical effect in 50% of the population, whether human or experimental animal), and LD_{50} is the median lethal dose (which produces death in 50% of experimental animals). The **ratio** LD_{50}/ED_{50} is the therapeutic index. Drugs that are relatively non-toxic have a high therapeutic index (LD_{50} much higher than ED_{50}), while the reverse is true of the more toxic drugs, such as digoxin (LD_{50} closer to ED_{50}). The slope of the dose–response curve is usually an indicator of the drug's toxicity – the lower the therapeutic index, the more steep the rise of the slope. In the example opposite, LD_{50} is about ten times higher than ED_{50}; the therapeutic index is sufficiently large.

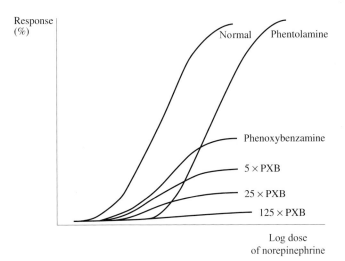

Figure 125. Competitive and non-competitive antagonism of norepinephrine effect on log dose–response curve.

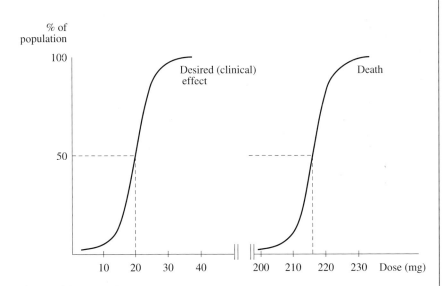

Figure 126. ED_{50}, LD_{50}.

4 Minimum alveolar concentration and lipid solubility

Minimum alveolar concentration (MAC) is defined as such a concentration of a volatile anaesthetic agent that produces **immobility in 50% of experimental animals** subjected to a standardized noxious stimulus. It resembles ED_{50} for intravenous drugs, and serves the same purpose: comparison of the potencies of various drugs. Potency of inhalational anaesthetic agents is usually directly proportional to their lipid solubility, although many exceptions exist. MAC is indirectly related to lipid solubility (the more potent a drug, the lower its MAC). Figure 127 illustrates this relationship. Both axes have logarithmic scales; the oil/gas partition coefficient is plotted on the x-axis against MAC in atmospheres on the y-axis. It can be seen that the points representing the position of individual agents lie close to a straight line. The product of MAC and solubility on this graph is about 2. The straight line seen on the graph is the result of double logarithmic transformation of a rectangular hyperbola, the shape that would depict the reciprocal relationship between MAC and lipid solubility on a linear scale. The logarithmic scales have the advantage of accommodating a wide range of numbers in a relatively small space.

MAC of nitrous oxide is above atmospheric, and its lipid solubility is very low. MACs for the other agents are given in oxygen for the upper line, and 66% nitrous oxide on the lower line. MAC is reduced by 60% by this concentration of nitrous oxide, as the effects are additive. This reduction is represented by the vertical arrows joining the corresponding points for each agent.

Notice that isoflurane and enflurane are one of the exceptions to the reciprocal relationship rule: isoflurane has a lower MAC (is more potent) than enflurane (1.15 v.s 1.68%), yet it has a slightly lower lipid solubility (91 v.s 96). The ascending order of the names from halothane at the lower end to nitrous oxide at the upper end applies to the minimum alveolar concentration but not to lipid solubility in the case of isoflurane and enflurane.

MAC is usually converted to percentage of atmospheric pressure, i.e. partial pressure. For instance, the MAC of halothane is 0.76% in 100% oxygen, or < 1%. The corresponding point for halothane is indeed slightly below 0.01 atm., or 1%.

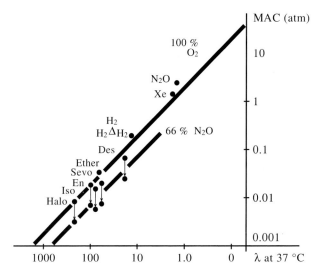

Figure 127. MAC and lipid solubility of volatile agents in 100% oxygen and in 66% nitrous oxide.

Receptor types, molecular action of anaesthetics

Receptors are molecules in the cell membrane whose function is to cause a response in target tissue after the binding of a specific ligand (a molecule for which the receptor has high affinity). The binding usually results in conformational change, and this triggers the response. Three types of receptors, the ligand – gated ion channel, the G-protein coupled receptor system, and the transmembrane enzymatic receptor, will be described here. It should be noted that the voltage – sensitive ion channel is not strictly speaking a receptor as it does not bind any molecules.

Multisubunit ligand – gated ion channel

Examples of this type are the nicotinic, GABA1 and glycine receptors. The macromolecule is a conical structure with the "thick" end protruding into the extracellular space. It is composed of four or more usually five subunits (it is a tetra- or pentamer). These subunits are called by the Greek letters α, β, γ, δ, and ϵ; a variant called the ρ type exists in the GABA1 receptor. Their structure is very similar to each other. Each subunit has four transmembrane domains called M1 to M4, where the protein crosses from extra- to intracellular or vice versa. The domains are shown opposite in Figure 128 as the grey rectangles. The M2 domain is involved in ligand (anaesthetic) binding. It can be seen that both the amino- and the carboxyl residue are extracellular; the amino residue is long, which forms the extracellular bulk mentioned above. The subunits are arranged in the tetra – or pentamer as shown in Figure 128, a cross section of the whole receptor structure at the level of the cell membrane. The receptor molecule is like a channel going through the membrane, with the subunits on the periphery of the channel. The transmembrane domains in each subunit are shown and it can be seen that they, too, are organised symmetrically inside the subunit.

G-protein coupled receptor

Examples of this type are the adrenergic receptor (adenyl cyclase), the phospholipase, and some muscarinic receptors. This receptor has seven transmembrane domains, with short amino and carboxyl residues on opposite sides of the cell membrane, as shown in Figure 129. In the vicinity of this peptide is the G-protein, the effector which converts guanosine triphosphate into guanosine diphosphate after receptor stimulation. Further aspects of this receptor are beyond the scope of this book.

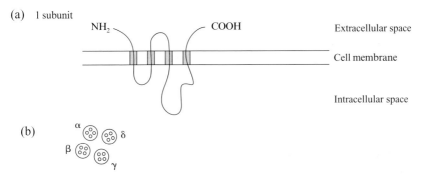

(a) 1 subunit

NH₂ ... COOH

Extracellular space

Cell membrane

Intracellular space

(b) α β γ δ

Figure 128. (a) Multisubunit ligand-gated ion channel.
(b) Cross-section of a tetramer (subunits α–δ).

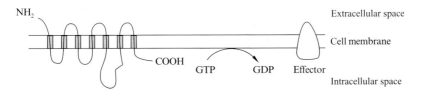

NH₂

COOH   GTP   GDP   Effector

Extracellular space

Cell membrane

Intracellular space

Figure 129. G-protein coupled receptor.

The transmembrane enzyme receptor

Examples of this type are the antinuclear factor, growth factor, neurotropic factor and others. These receptors are protein kinases mostly. As shown in Figure 130, the ligand binds to the extracellular receptor site; this produces a conformational change at the intracellular site with the result that the intra-cellular process is catalysed at a much faster rate.

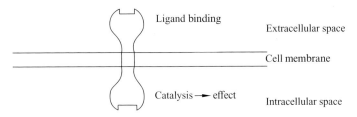

Figure 130. Receptor as enzyme.

Context-sensitive half-time

This concept was developed to describe drug elimination after an intravenous infusion, designed to produce a steady plasma concentration of a drug, is discontinued. Drugs which depend on the liver or kidneys for their elimination demonstrate this phenomenon. In practice, this encompasses all hypnotic drugs and opioids used in total intravenous anaesthesia, with the exception of remifentanil, which is eliminated from the body by tissue and plasma esterases. Half-time is the time required for the drug concentration to halve. Recovery cannot be expected before the plasma concentration decreases below 50% or the clinically effective concentration.

The half-time is context sensitive because **drug elimination depends on the duration** of infusion. To understand it, consider the three-compartment pharmacological model, consisting of the central compartment-C_1-(the intravascular space) and two peripheral compartments, one which equilibrates with the central compartment fairly rapidly-C_2-(well perfused tissues such as the brain) and the other which equilibrates more slowly because of poorer perfusion-C_3-(fat). The rich or poor perfusion is illustrated in the figures opposite by a wide or narrow band connecting the compartments.

After a **short duration infusion**, the peripheral compartments have not yet reached equilibrium with the central compartment (see Figure 131). Therefore, after the infusion is discontinued, plasma concentration declines fairly rapidly as the drug continues to redistribute into the peripheral compartments, until equilibrium is reached at a lower plasma concentration. Because redistribution is faster that elimination, context-sensitive half-time in this situation is closer to the redistribution half-life.

After a **prolonged infusion**, the peripheral compartments reached equilibrium with the central compartment and drug concentration is the same in all three (steady state), as shown in Figure 132. On discontinuing the infusion, plasma concentration can only decline by drug elimination from the central compartment via liver or kidneys. As the drug is being eliminated, more drug is moved from the peripheral compartments into the central compartment, adding to the drug load to be eliminated. Hence the context-sensitive half-time in this situation is close to elimination half-life.

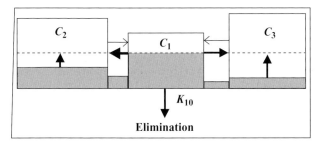

C_1 central compartment

C_2, C_3 peripheral compartments

Figure 131. Drug levels in three compartments after a short infusion.

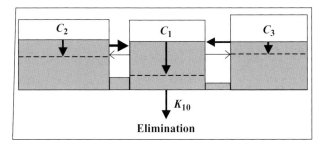

Figure 132. Drug levels in three compartments after a prolonged infusion.

Figure 133 shows the observed decline of plasma alfentanil concentration after an infusion of 10-minute and 3-hour duration. Although the initial plasma concentration is the same (100 ng/ml), the decline clearly varies for different duration of the infusion. The half-time after the 3-hour infusion is four times greater.

Context-sensitive half-time for various anaesthetic drugs is plotted in Figure 134 (short infusion) and 135 (prolonged infusion). Remifentanil, which has a half-time of 3 minutes, independent of duration of infusion, is included for comparison. For other drugs, context-sensitive half-time increases more or less in the form of a sigmoid curve, until after several hours a steady state is reached. The point at which the context-sensitive half-time reaches a plateau depends on the volume of distribution of the drug in all three compartments: the larger the V_D, the longer it takes to reach steady state. Notice that the line for fentanyl intersects the alfentanil and thiopentone line. This, in practice, means that after a short infusion of up to 2 hours, fentanyl will be cleared more rapidly than alfentanil, but the reverse is true when the duration of infusion is longer than 2 hours. This is because of the difference between the redistribution and elimination half-life of the two drugs. Because of its high lipid solubility, context-sensitive half-time for fentanyl has not reached a plateau even after 12 hours, whereas the other drugs have reached, or are near, a plateau after 3 hours. Therefore, after a prolonged infusion, fentanyl ends up with the slowest elimination of the drugs illustrated in the drawing.

In practice, context-sensitive half-time may be expressed in the form of a 'fraction', with the 'redistribution' half-time (concerning a short infusion of 10 minutes) in the 'nominator' and 'elimination' half-time (concerning a prolonged infusion of 3 hours) in the 'denominator'. Thus remifentanil has a context sensitive half-time of 3/3, alfentanil 10/40 and fentanyl 3/70. Pharmacokinetic data for fentanyl are inconsistent and other values may be found in different sources.

Devices for target-controlled infusion use the model of context-sensitive half-time to predict the decline in plasma concentration after the infusion is stopped. Therefore, it is possible to calculate the expected time to 'waking up' – effectively to a subhypnotic plasma concentration. Propofol, with a context sensitive half-time of 5/9, is a suitable drug for total intravenous anaesthesia. Even after a 12-hour infusion the half-time is 18 minutes. Thiopentone with a context sensitive half-time of 4/85 is not suitable for continuous infusion where rapid wakefulness is desired after stopping the sedation. Thiopentone may still be used in specific indications, for instance status epilepticus, for its pharmacodynamic properties.

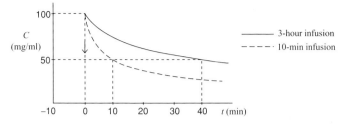

Figure 133. Plasma alfentanil concentration after short and long infusion.

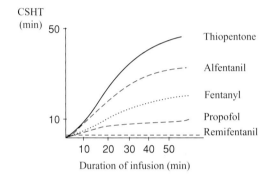

Figure 134. Context-sensitive half-time after short infusion.

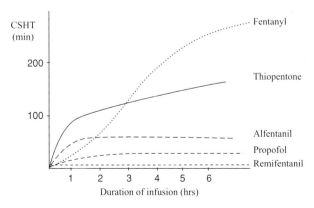

Figure 135. Context-sensitive half-time after prolonged infusion.

Further Reading

Kenny, G., Davis, P. D. *Basic Physics and Measurement in Anaesthesia*. Butterworth Heinemann, 2003.

Miller, R. D. *Anaesthesia*. Edinburgh: Churchill Livingstone, 2000.

Peck, T. E., Williams, M. *Pharmacology for Anaesthesia and Intensive Care*. Greenwich Medical Media, 2000.

Mepleson, W. W. Fifty years after reflections on The elimination of rebreathing in various semi-closed anaesthetic systems. *Br. J. Anaesth*. 2004; 93: 319–21.

Pinnock, C., Lim, T., Smith, T. *Fundamentals of Anaesthesia*. Greenwich Medical Media, 2002.

Prys-Roberts, C. *The Circulation in Anaesthesia*. Oxford: Blackwell, 1980.

Scurr, C., Feldman, S. *Scientific Foundations of Anaesthesia*. Oxford: Butterworth-Heinemann.

www.frca.co.uk.

INDEX

Page references in *italic* indicate figures.